Lactogenic Diet Book

Quick, Easy & Delicious Lactogenic Recipes for Breasting Mums

BY: Ivy Hope

Copyright © 2021 by Ivy Hope

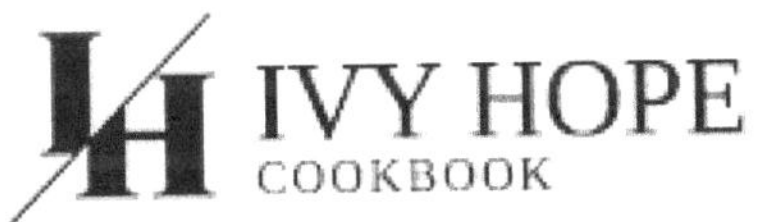

Copyright/License Page

Please don't reproduce this book. It means you are not allowed to make any type of copy (print or electronic), sell, publish, disseminate or distribute. Only people who have written permission from the author are allowed to do so.

This book is written by the author taking all precautions that the content is true and helpful. However, the reader needs to be careful about his/her action. If anything happens due to the reader's actions the author won't be taken as responsible.

Table of Contents

Introduction

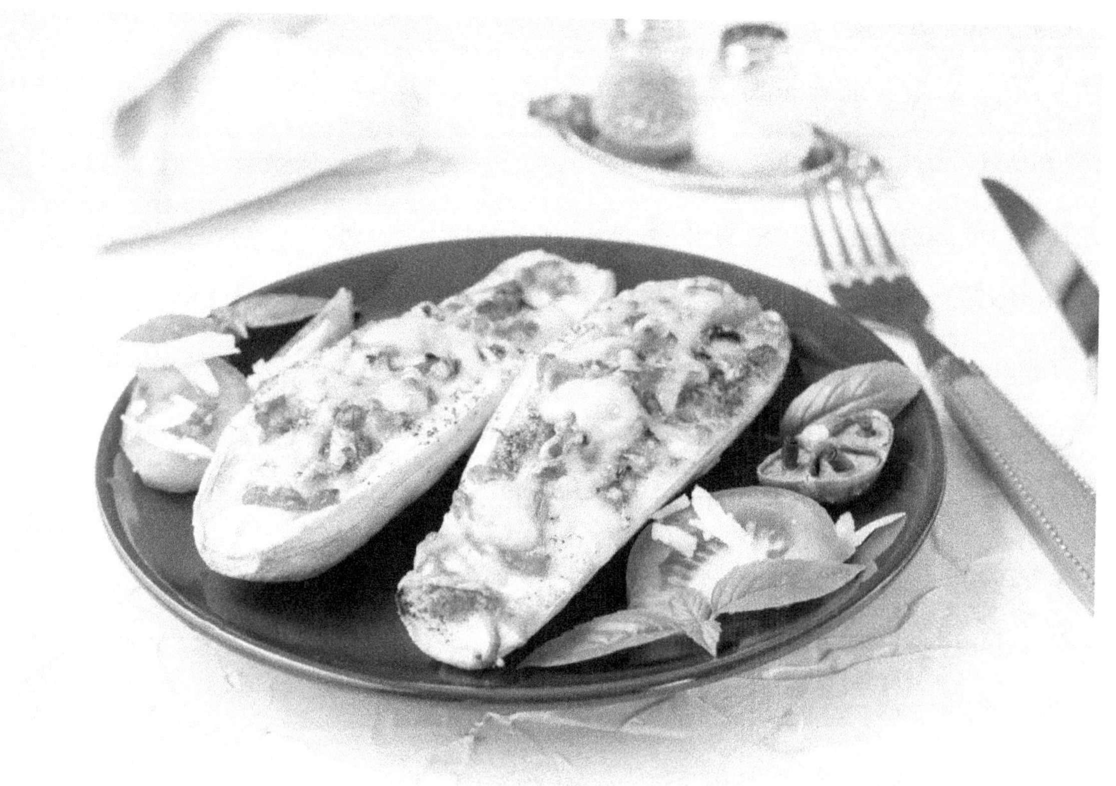

Lactogenic diets have been proven to reduce body fat content without increasing insulin levels, thus preventing weight regain after fasting. Lactogens also help promote healthy cholesterol levels and blood sugar regulation.

The Lactogenic diet has been reported to reduce the number of carbohydrates consumed from anywhere between 10-25%. It is also reported to increase insulin production, which could mean that the diet could potentially cause weight loss.

The Lactogenic diet is also known to induce the production of growth hormones. Growth hormone is a hormone produced by the pituitary gland that stimulates tissue repair, tissue growth, and increases muscle mass. This happens at around a half-hour after consuming carbohydrates, after which the fat content in your body starts to grow, most likely since carbohydrates are no longer being consumed. Testosterone and several other hormones are also released. In short, eating carbohydrates results in more fat being burned than other foods, which is why it is better to eat high-calorie foods low in carbohydrate content.

This book contains 50 delicious lactogenic recipes that have been carefully selected for you to enjoy.

Happy cooking!

Chapter 1: Breakfast recipes

Simple Baked Oatmeal

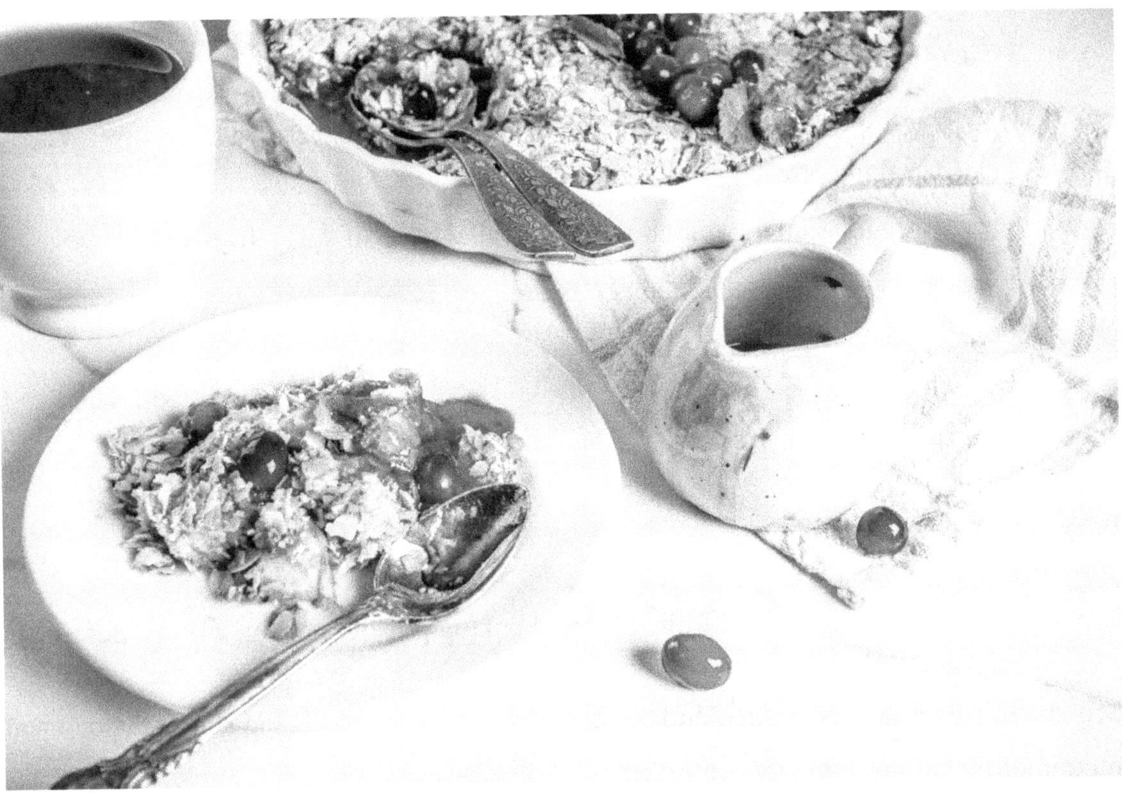

Simple Baked Oatmeal is a delicious dish that's as easy to make as it is to put away for leftovers! Combine oats with eggs, water, and other ingredients like milk, brown sugar, or honey. Or mix in blueberries or any fruit you prefer to customize your dish.

Serving size: 10

Cooking time: 25 minutes

Ingredients:

- 4 cups of quick-cooking or old-fashioned oats
- 1 cup of light brown sugar
- 2/3 cup or more of dried cranberries, raisins 2-3 of walnuts, pecans
- 2 tsp. of baking powder
- 3 cups of regular milk, almond milk, soy milk 1 cup of sugar-free applesauce
- 4 of unsalted butter, melted and set aside
- 2 large eggs, beaten and set aside

Instructions:

Preheat your oven to 375°F.

Mix the oats, brown sugar, dried fruit, nuts, and baking powder in a large bowl. Set aside.

Mix the milk, applesauce, butter, and beaten eggs in another bowl, and add to the oatmeal mixture. Mix until thoroughly combined.

Grease ramekins, 8-inch pans or any other baking dish of your choice. Ramekins make it easier to portion the oatmeal, so using them is highly recommended. Use medium to large sized ramekins for this recipe.

Spoon or pour the oatmeal into the baking dish of your choice. Bake for 15-25 minutes until slightly golden brown and cooked through.

Serve warm with extra fruits or Greek yogurt.

Breakfast Tomato and Eggs

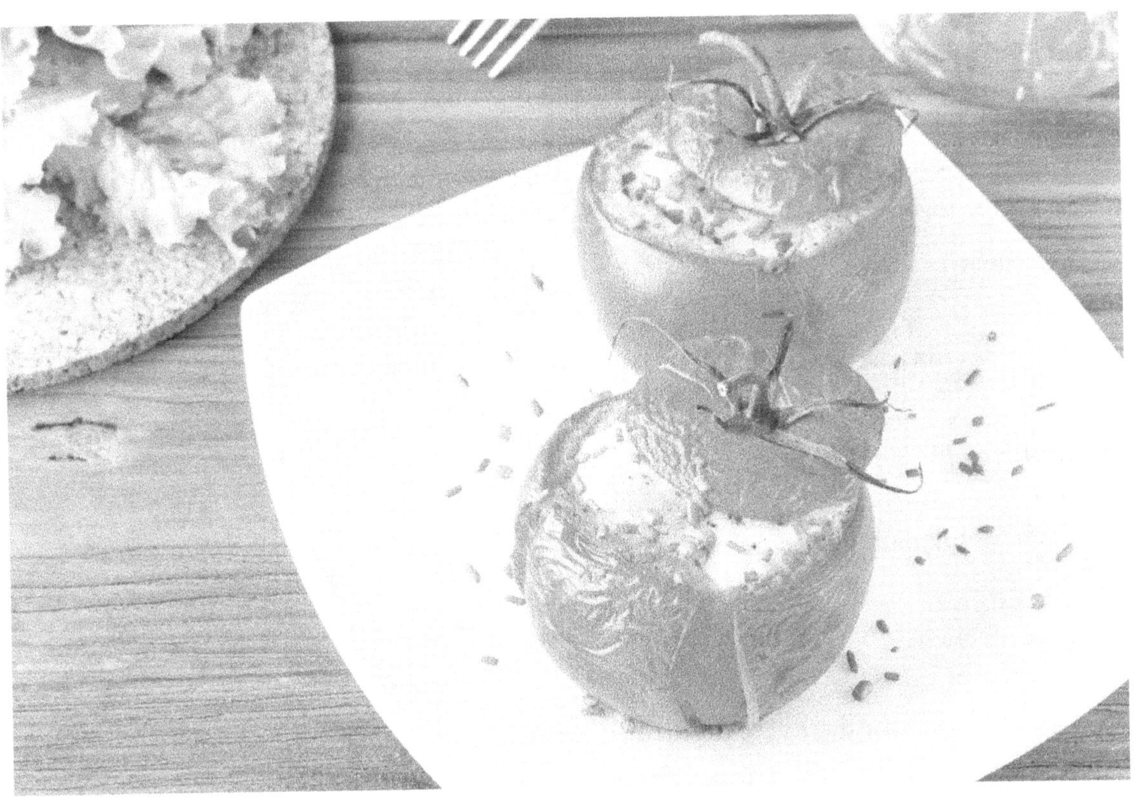

Packed with protein, vitamins, and antioxidants, this breakfast meal provides a quick way to start your day.

This dish is also straightforward to make, and it's a dish that the whole family can enjoy, even your picky eaters! It's perfect for those mornings when you're in a rush but still want something satisfying to eat before you head out the door.

Serving size: 2

Cooking time: 30 minutes

Ingredients:

- 2 eggs
- 2 tomatoes
- Salt and black pepper to taste
- 1 tsp. parsley, finely chopped

Instructions:

Cut tomatoes tops, scoop flesh, and arrange them on a lined baking sheet.

Crack an egg in each tomato.

Season with salt and pepper.

Introduce them in the oven at 300°F and bake for 30 minutes

Take tomatoes out of the oven, divide between plates, season with more salt and pepper, sprinkle parsley at the end, and serve.

Enjoy!

Plantain Pancakes

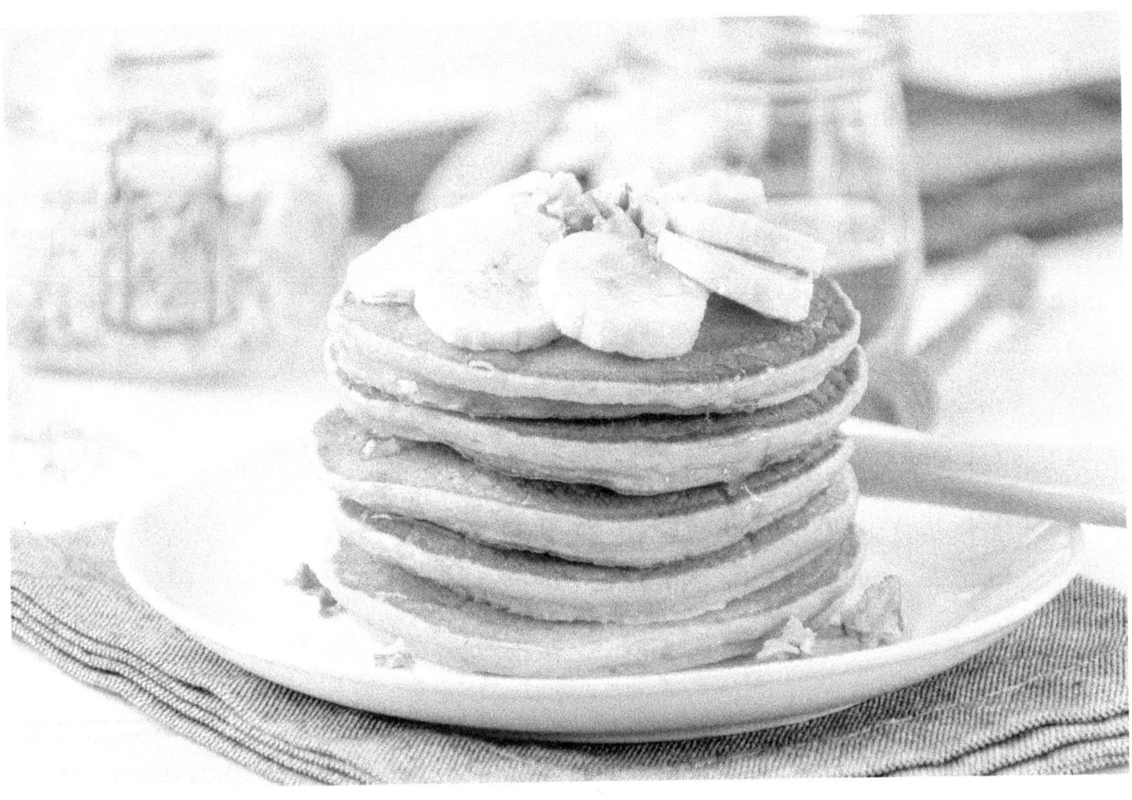

Plantain pancakes are just delicious! They're so soft and moist, and they hold up to all kinds of tastiness. Plantain pancakes are a great vegan option for those who don't want to eat eggs or dairy in their diet. This gluten-free recipe is also high in fiber and protein.

Serving size: 4

Cooking time: 5 minutes

Ingredients:

- 3 eggs
- ¼ cup coconut flour
- ¼ cup coconut water
- 1 tsp. coconut oil
- ½ plantain, peeled and chopped
- ¼ tsp. baking soda
- ¼ tsp. cream of tartar
- A pinch of salt
- ¼ tsp. chai spice
- 1 tbsp. shaved coconut, toasted for serving
- 1 tbsp. coconut milk for serving

Instructions:

In your food processor, mix eggs with a pinch of salt, coconut water and flour, plantain, cream of tartar, baking soda, and chai spice. Blend well.

Heat up a pan with the coconut oil over medium heat, add ¼ cup pancake batter, spread evenly, cook until it becomes golden, flip pancake and cook for one minute and transfer to a plate.

Serve pancakes with shaved coconut and coconut milk.

Sweet Potato Waffles

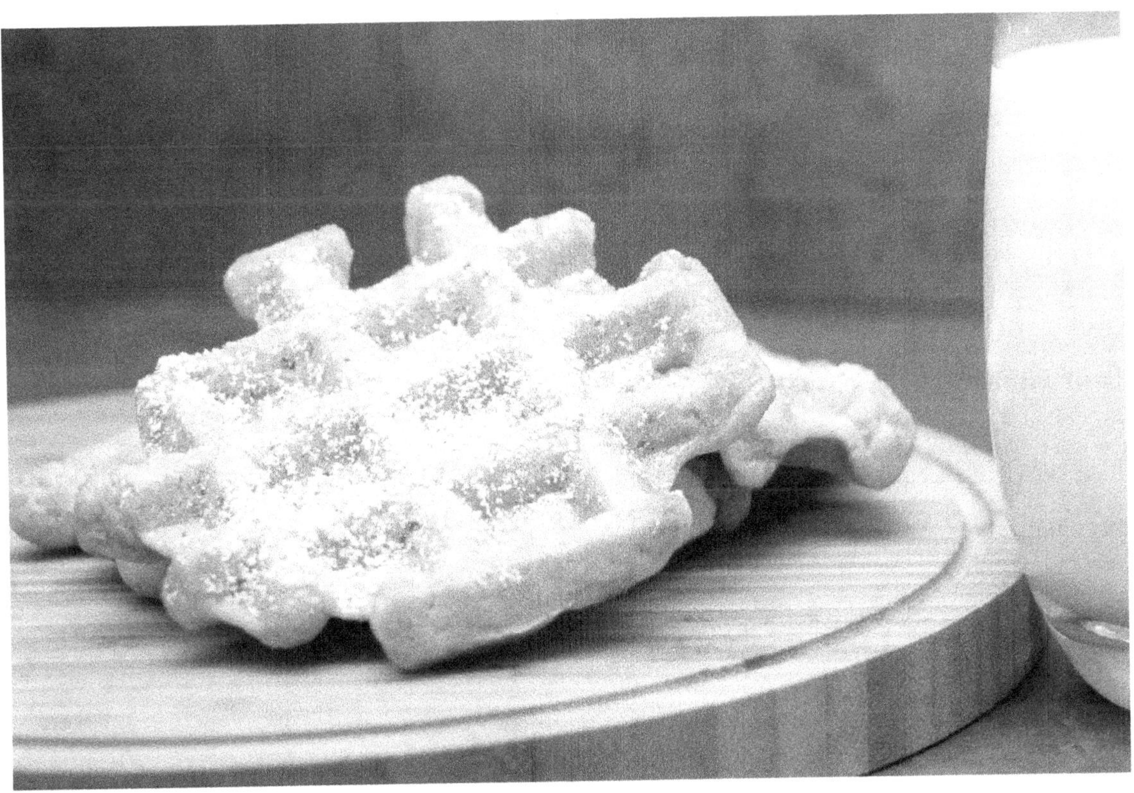

These waffles, in particular, are crispy on the outside and fluffy inside with just the right amount of sweetness and spice to get your morning off to a fantastic start.

Serving size: 4

Cooking time: 10 minutes

Ingredients:

- 2 sweet potatoes, peeled and finely grated
- 2 tbsp. melted coconut oil
- 3 eggs
- 1 tsp. cinnamon powder
- ½ tsp. nutmeg, ground
- Some apple sauce for serving

Instructions:

In a bowl, mix eggs with sweet potatoes, coconut oil, cinnamon, and nutmeg and whisk very well.

Cook waffles in your waffle iron, arrange them on plates, and serve with apple sauce drizzled on top.

Orange and Dates Granola

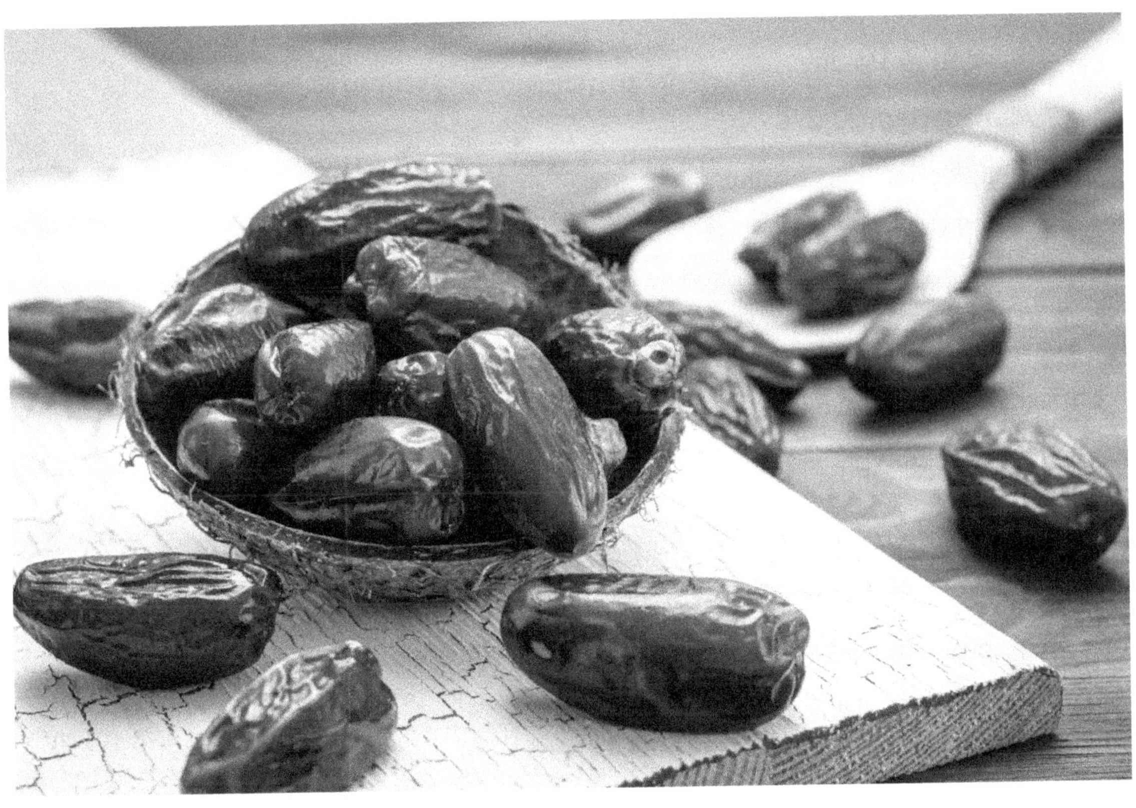

If you have any old dates in the back cupboard, this is an excellent way to use them and transform them into something delicious.

This tasty recipe can be made in minutes, and it provides the perfect healthy breakfast. It's so versatile that you can also experiment with other nuts or seeds to get various textures.

Serving size: 6

Cooking time: 15 minutes

Ingredients:

- 5 oz. dates, soaked in hot water
- Juice from 1 orange
- ½ orange grated rind
- 1 cup desiccated coconut
- ½ cup silvered almonds
- ½ cup pumpkin seeds
- ½ cup linseeds
- ½ cup sesame seeds
- Almond milk for serving

Instructions:

In a bowl, mix almonds with orange rind, orange juice, linseeds, and coconut, pumpkin, and sesame seeds, and stir well.

Drain dates, add them to your food processor, and blend well.

Add this paste to almonds, mix and stir well again.

Spread this on a lined baking sheet, introduce it in the oven at 350°F and bake for 15 minutes, stirring every 4 minutes.

Take granola out of the oven, leave aside to cool down a bit and then serve with almond milk.

Spinach Frittata

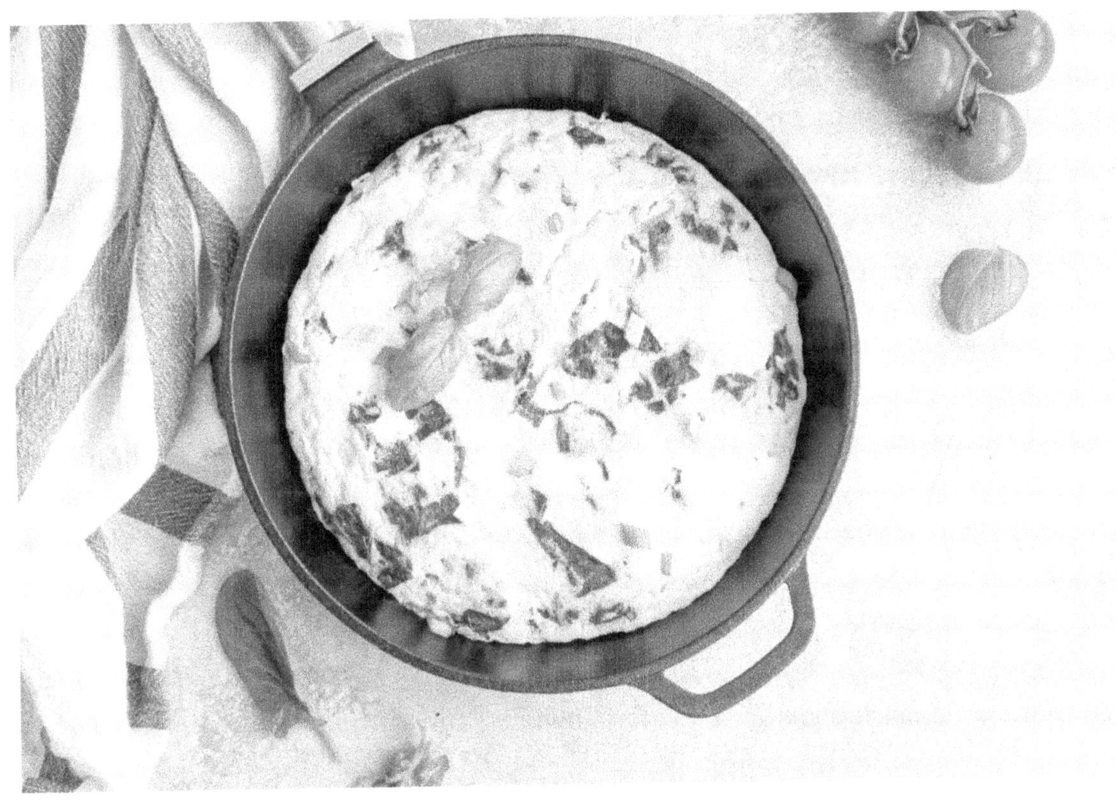

This recipe is not only a delicious egg dish but also an excellent way to get in your leafy greens. The frittata consists of spinach, eggs, ricotta cheese, Parmesan cheese, and garlic. It is oven-baked with some bacon and topped off with chives.

Serving size: 4

Cooking time: 25 minutes

Ingredients:

- ½ lb. sausage, ground
- 2 tbsp. ghee
- 1 cup mushrooms, thinly sliced
- 1 cup spinach leaves, chopped
- 10 eggs, whisked
- 1 small yellow onion, finely chopped
- Salt and black pepper to taste

Instructions:

Heat a pan with the ghee over medium-high heat, add onion, stir and cook until it browns.

Add sausage, stir and also cook until it browns.

Add spinach and mushrooms and cook for 4 minutes, stirring from time to time.

Take the pan off the heat, add eggs, spread evenly, introduce frittata in the oven at 150°F and bake for 20 minutes

Take frittata out of the oven, leave it aside for a few moments to cool down, cut, arrange on plates and serve.

Maple Nut Porridge

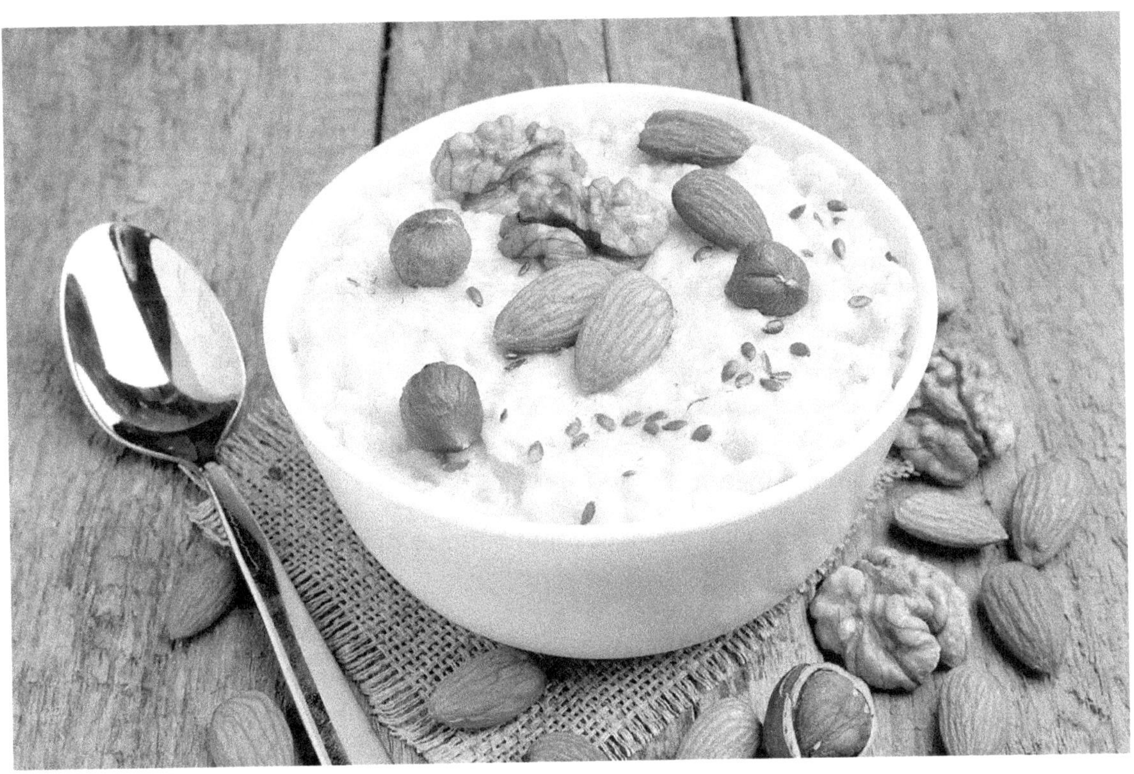

This maple nut porridge is the best and easiest recipe for anyone looking to start their morning off with a good breakfast. It's not too sweet and has a good mix of crunchy carbohydrates and healthy fats you will enjoy every time. If you want to eat something new and tasty, then you should consider trying this porridge!

Serving size: 4

Cooking time: 5 minutes

Ingredients:

- ½ cup pecans, soaked
- ¾ cup of hot water
- 1 peeled and chopped banana
- ½ tsp. cinnamon
- A pinch of salt
- 2 tsp. maple syrup
- 2 tbsp. coconut butter

Instructions:

Mix pecans with maple syrup, cinnamon, coconut butter, a pinch of salt, water, and banana in the food processor and mix well.

Transfer the mixture to a pan,

Heat the pan over medium heat and cook until it thickens and pour into a bowl and serve!

Turkey Breakfast Sandwich

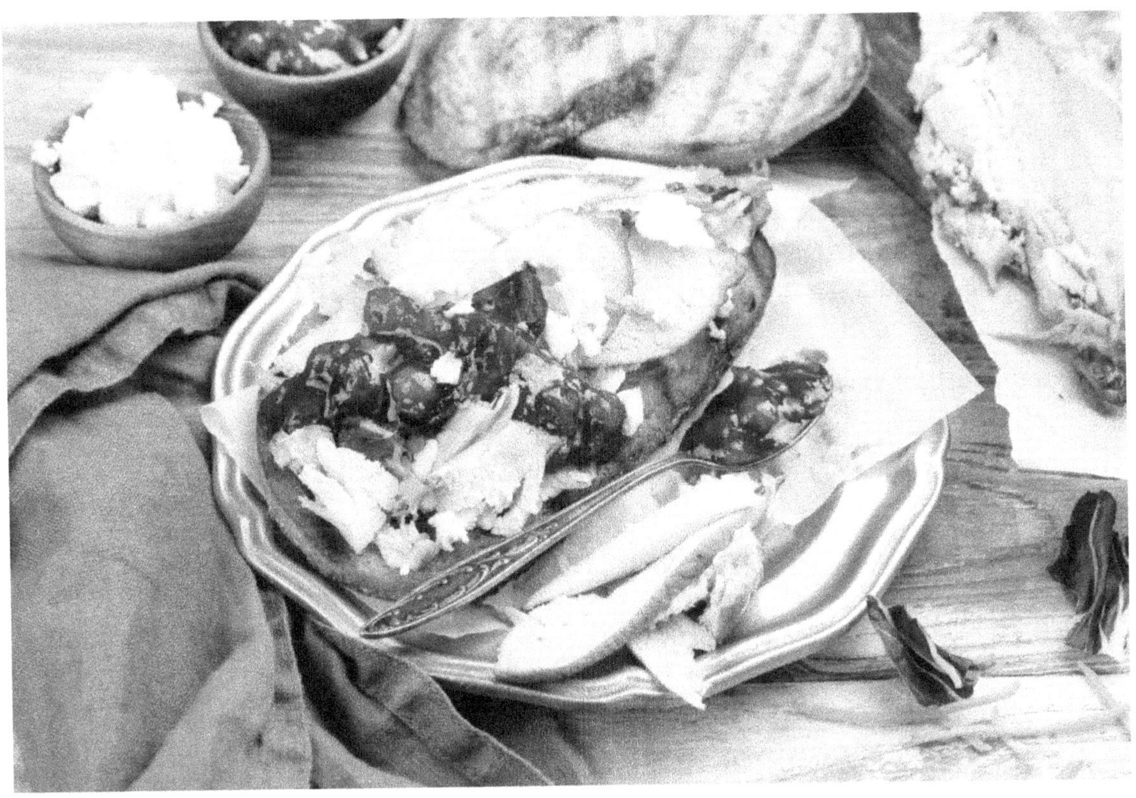

Whether you're in the mood for a quick breakfast or looking for a hearty afternoon snack, this is the perfect sandwich. It has all the flavors of your favorite meal. Turkey, stuffing, and cranberry sauce.

No other sandwich will taste this good! Just wait and see!

Serving size: 1

Cooking time: 0 minutes

Ingredients:

- 2 oz. turkey meat, roasted and thinly sliced
- 2 tbsp. pecans, toasted and chopped
- 2 oz. Brie cheese, sliced
- 2 slices sourdough bread
- 2 tbsp. cranberry chutney
- ¼ cup arugula

Instructions:

In a bowl, mix pecans with chutney and stir well.

Spread this on a bread slice, add turkey slices, brie cheese, and arugula and top with the other bread slice.

Serve right away.

Chicken Liver Breakfast Spread

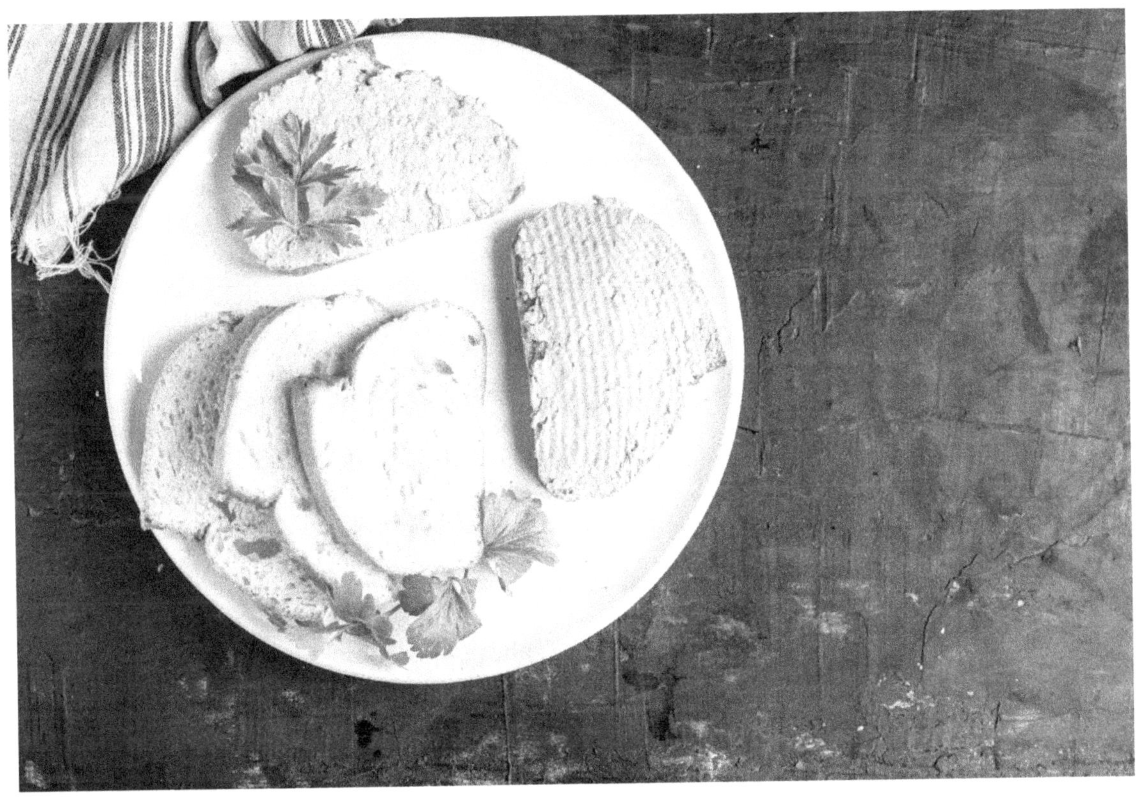

A delicious and healthy spread will energize your morning and promote brain health. Serve this healthy chicken liver breakfast spread with some whole grain toast or crackers! It's a perfect vehicle for sweeter breakfasts.

Serving size: 2

Cooking time: 10 minutes

Ingredients:

- 1 tsp. olive oil
- ¾ lb. chicken livers
- 1 yellow onion, chopped
- ¼ cup water
- 1 bay leaf
- 2 anchovies
- 1 tbsp. capers
- 1 tbsp. ghee
- A pinch of salt and black pepper

Instructions:

Put the olive oil in your instant pot, add onion, salt, pepper, chicken livers, water, and the bay leaf, stir, cover, and cook on high for 10 minutes.

Discard bay leaf, add anchovies, capers, and ghee, and pulse everything using your immersion blender.

Add salt and pepper, blend again, divide into bowls and serve for breakfast.

Mushroom Spread

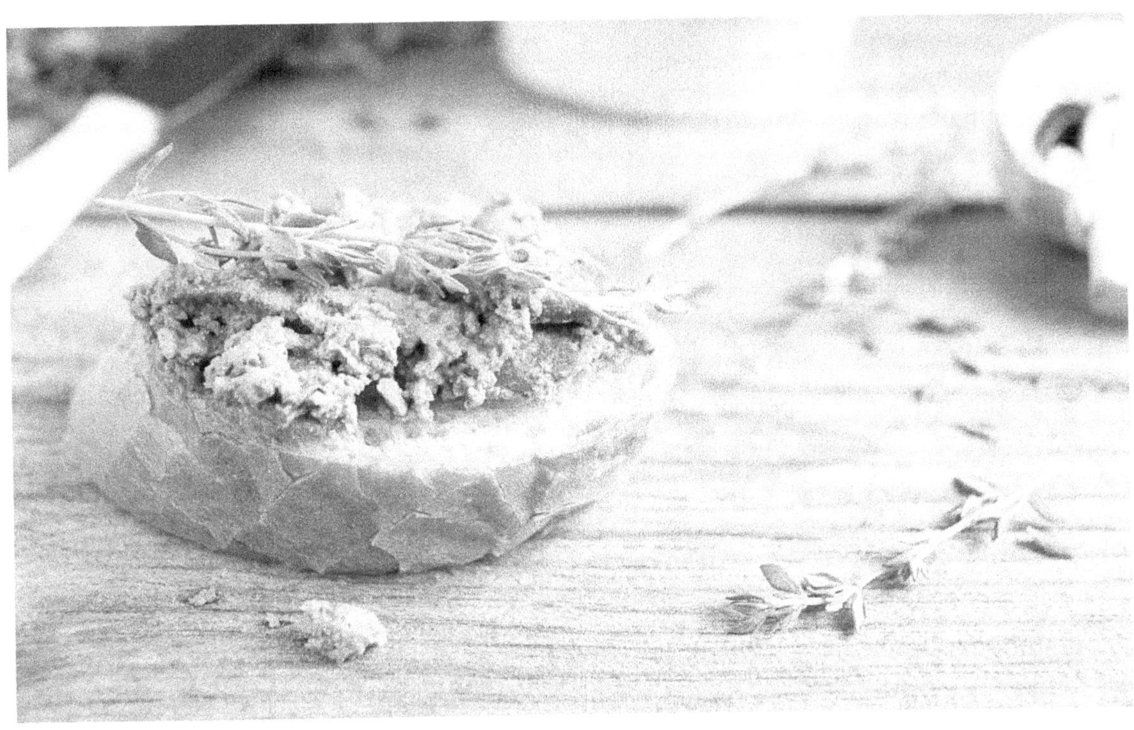

The most important part of making an excellent mushroom spread is using a perfect sour cream. If you're looking for something with more flavor, try substituting Greek yogurt for sour cream.

Mushrooms make a great breakfast because they're easy to make and nutritious.

Serving size: 2

Cooking time: 14 minutes

Ingredients:

- 1 oz. porcini mushrooms, dried
- 1 lb. button mushrooms, sliced
- 1 cup hot water
- 1 tbsp. ghee
- 1 tbsp. olive oil
- 1 shallot, chopped
- ¼ cup cold water
- A pinch of salt and pepper
- 1 bay leaf

Instructions:

Put porcini mushrooms in a bowl, add 1 cup hot water and leave aside for now.

Set your instant pot on sauté mode, add ghee, and oil and heat it.

Add shallot, stir and sauté for 2 minutes

Add porcini mushrooms and their liquid, fresh mushrooms, cold, salt, pepper, and bay leaf, stir, cover, and cook on high for 12 minutes.

Discard bay leaf and some of the liquid and blend mushrooms mix using an immersion blender.

Transfer to small bowls and serve as a breakfast spread.

Breakfast Chia Pudding

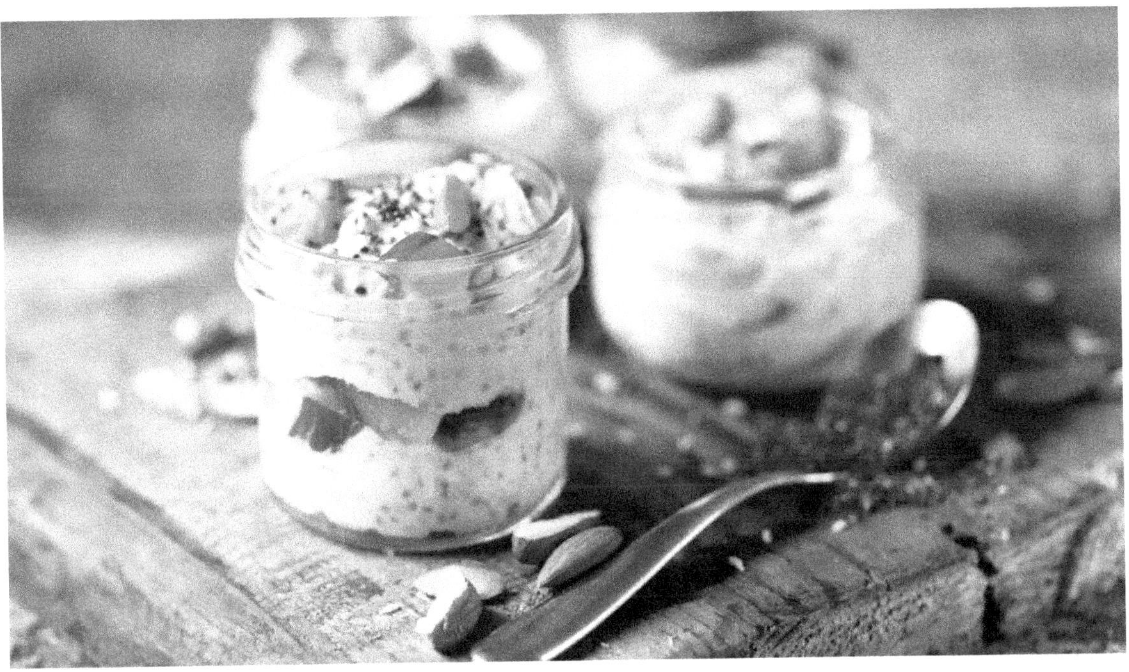

The chia seed is a powerhouse of nutrients and a cinch to make. These healing seeds are small enough to fit in any diet without being overpowering, and they're so easy to find in any grocery store. As long as you have water at the ready, you can prepare this breakfast guaranteed to satisfy.

Serving size: 2

Cooking time: 3 minutes

Ingredients:

- ½ cup chia seeds
- 2 cups almond milk
- ¼ cup almonds
- ¼ cup coconut, shredded
- 4 tsp. sugar

Instructions:

Put chia seeds in your instant pot.

Add milk, almonds, and coconut flakes, stir, cover, and cook at high for 3 minutes.

Release the pressure quickly, divide the pudding between bowls, top each with a teaspoon of sugar and serve.

Breakfast Sweet Potatoes

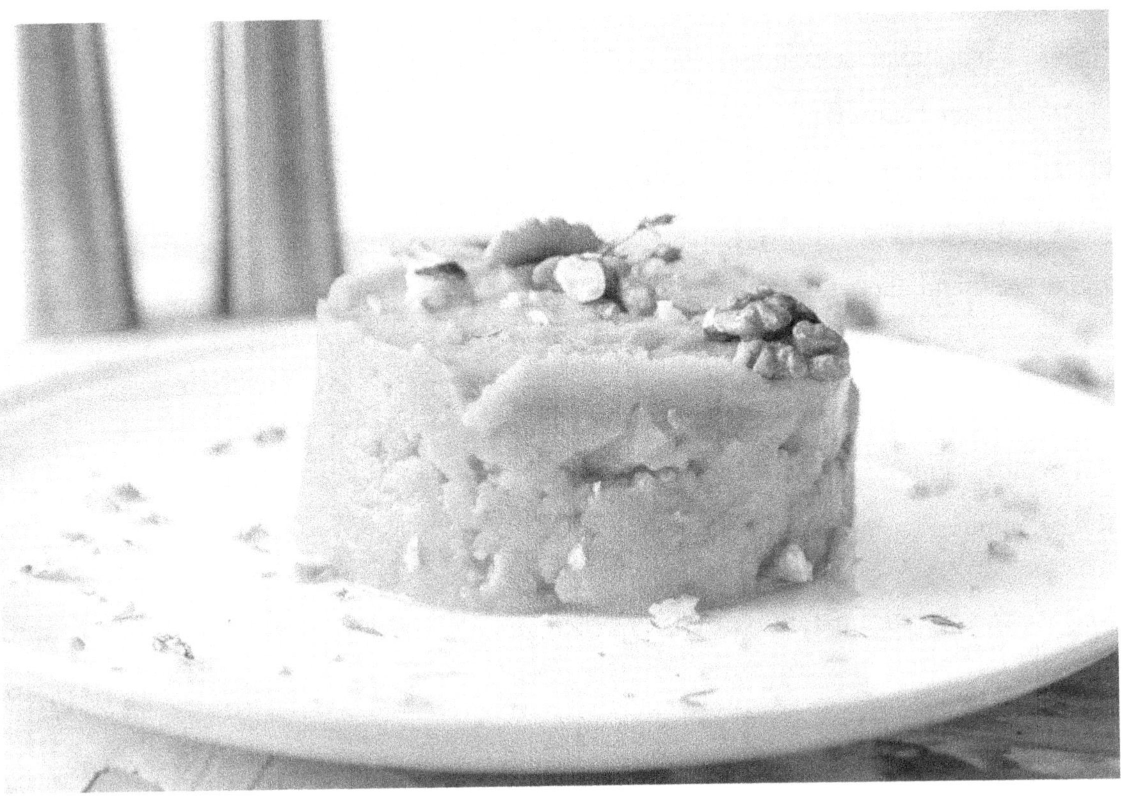

It's a simple dish that is so easy to make and is not at all time-consuming. It only takes a few minutes, and you can combine it with anything you want for breakfast. Breakfast sweet potatoes are quick, easy, and you can add just about anything you want.

Serving size: 2

Cooking time: 10 minutes

Ingredients:

- 4 sweet potatoes
- 2 tsp. Italian seasoning
- 1 tbsp. bacon fat
- 1 cup chives, chopped for serving.
- Water
- Salt and pepper to taste

Instructions:

Put potatoes in your instant pot, add water to cover them, cover the pot and cook at high for 10 minutes.

Release the pressure naturally, transfer potatoes to a working surface and leave them to cool down.

Peel potatoes, transfer them to a bowl and mash them a bit with a fork.

Set your instant pot on sauté mode, add bacon fat and heat up.

Add potatoes, seasoning, salt and pepper to the taste, stir, cover the pot and cook at high for 1 minute.

Release the pressure quickly, stir potatoes again, divide them between plates and serve with chives sprinkled on top.

Different Eggs Breakfast

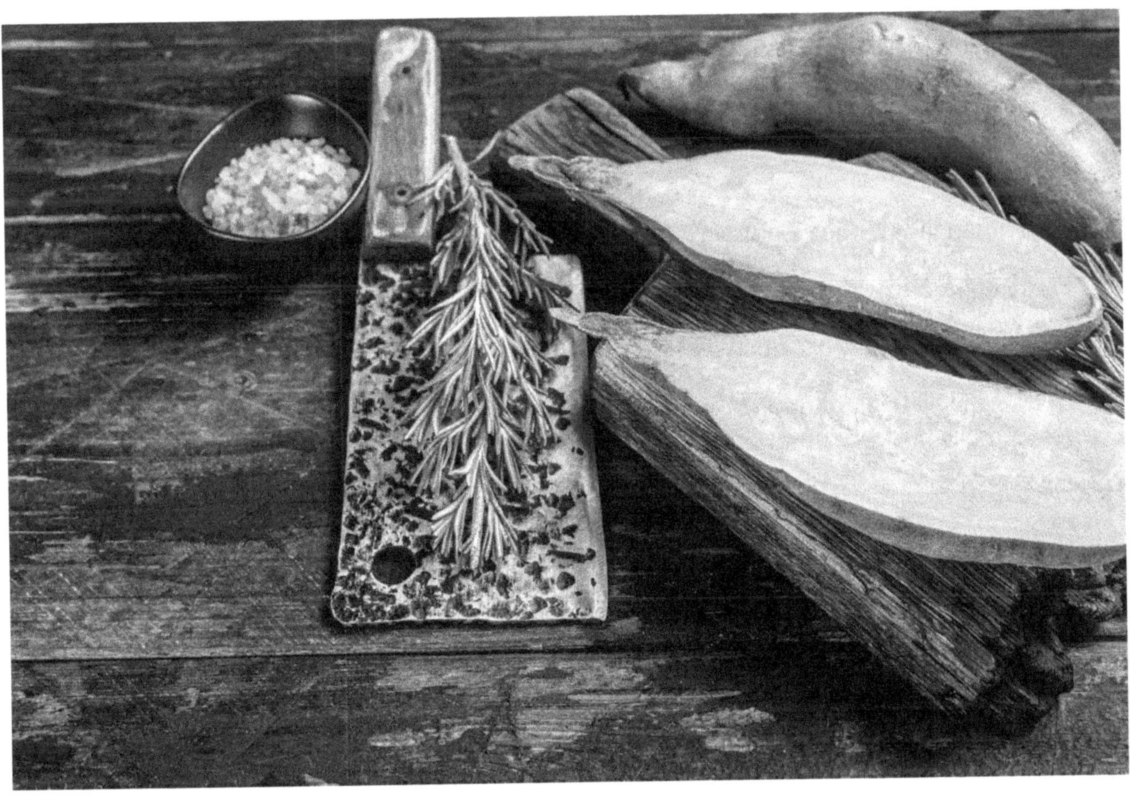

It is easy to make but can also be made in advance and conveniently stored at room temperature for several days without losing its freshness.

Serving size: 2

Cooking time: 5 minutes

Ingredients:

- 2 tbsp. olive oil
- 1 cup water
- 1 cup sweet potatoes, cubed
- 2 eggs
- 1 jalapeno pepper, chopped
- ½ cup yellow onion, chopped
- 1 tbsp. cilantro, chopped
- A pinch of salt and black pepper

Instructions:

Put 1 cup water in your instant pot, add the steamer basket, place cubed potatoes inside, cover, and cook on high for 3 minutes and transfer to a bowl.

Take the steamer basket out, clean the instant pot, add the oil and set the pot on sauté mode.

Add onion, jalapeno and return potato cubes, stir and sauté for a couple of minutes.

Crack eggs, season with a pinch of salt, black pepper and sprinkle cilantro.

Stir gently, cover and cook on high for 2 minutes.

Divide this breakfast mix between plates and serve.

Porridge

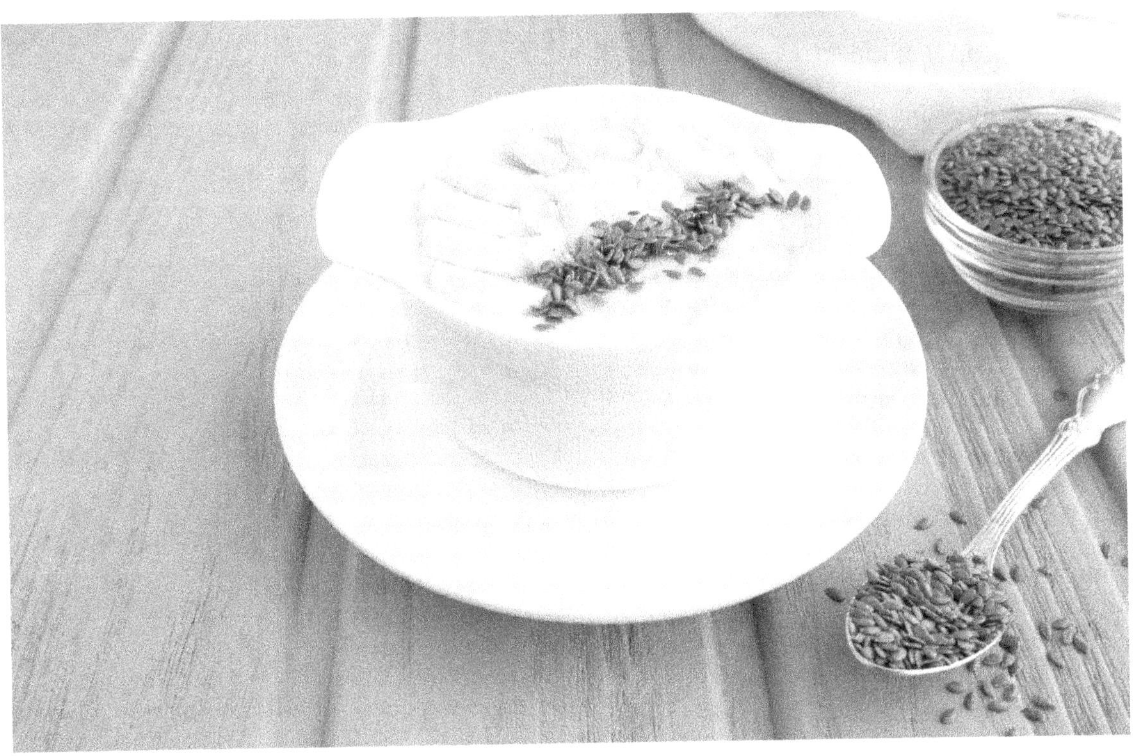

Sugar, salt, and flour are staples in most kitchens. They bring flavor and texture to your meals and make it easier to cook everything from rice to biscuits. But there is one ingredient that is so much more than just a culinary staple: it's nearly impossible to have a healthy diet without porridge.

Serving size: 3

Cooking time: 6 minutes

Ingredients:

- 1 big plantain; peeled and mashed
- ¼ cup flax meal
- 2 cups coconut milk
- 3/4 cup almond meal
- 1 tsp. cinnamon; powder
- A pinch of cloves; ground
- ½ tsp. ginger powder
- A pinch of nutmeg; ground
- Maple syrup for serving
- Some unsweetened coconut flakes for serving

Instructions:

In a small pan, mix plantain with flax meal, almond meal, coconut milk, cinnamon, cloves, ginger and nutmeg, stir well, bring to a simmer over medium heat and cook for about 6 minutes.

Divide your porridge into bowls, top with coconut flakes and maple syrup and serve.

Apple Pancakes

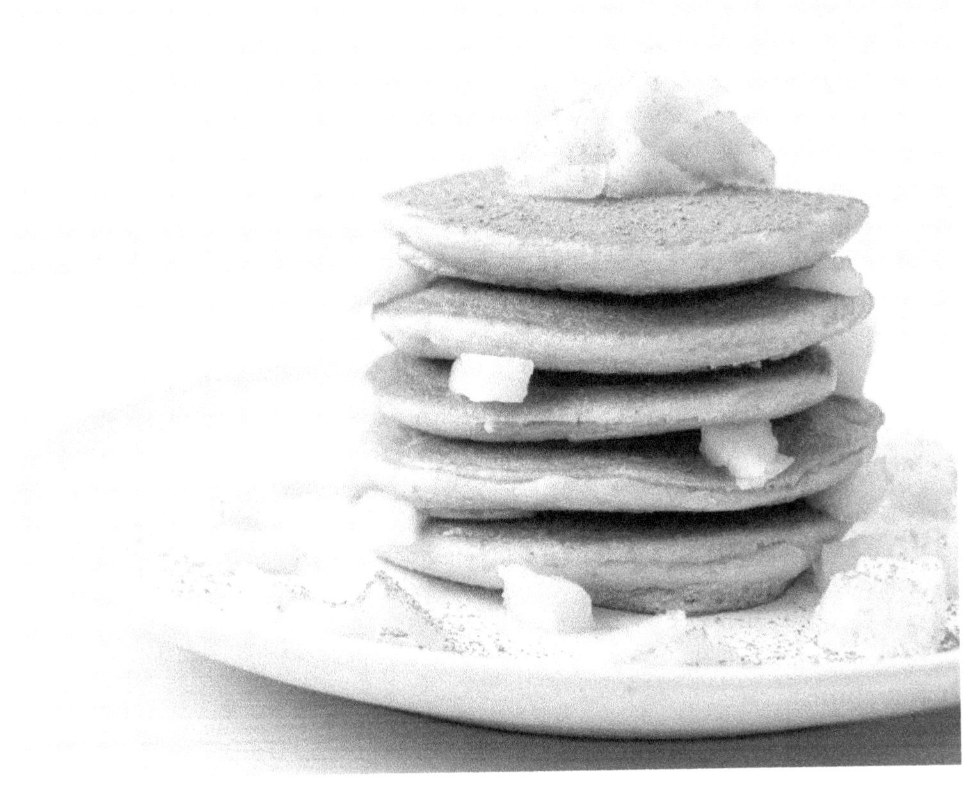

Apple Pancakes are easy to make, and they taste outstanding. And let's be honest, making pancakes never tasted this good before.

They're so versatile, too. They can work as a meal for breakfast or brunch with a side of bacon (or sausage!), a snack, or a dessert with ice cream.

Serving size: 18

Cooking time: 5 minutes

Ingredients:

- 2 cups apples; peeled, cored and chopped
- 1 tbsp. coconut oil
- 4 eggs
- 2 tsp. cinnamon powder
- 2 tbsp. honey
- 1 cup almond milk+ 3 tablespoons
- 1 tsp. vanilla extract
- ½ cup coconut flour
- A pinch of nutmeg
- ½ tsp. baking soda
- 3 tbsp. ghee
- 2 tbsp. maple syrup

Instructions:

Heat a pan with 1 tbsp. oil over medium heat, add apples and cinnamon, stir and cook for 5 minutes.

In a bowl, whisk eggs with vanilla, 1 cup milk, honey, baking soda, coconut flour and nutmeg and whisk. Add apples and the rest of the almond milk and stir again well.

Heat a pan with the ghee over medium-high heat, pour some of the pancake batter, spread, cook until it's done on one side, flip, cook on the other side as well and transfer to a plate.

Repeat with the rest of the batter and serve your pancakes with maple syrup on top.

Ham and Mushroom Breakfast

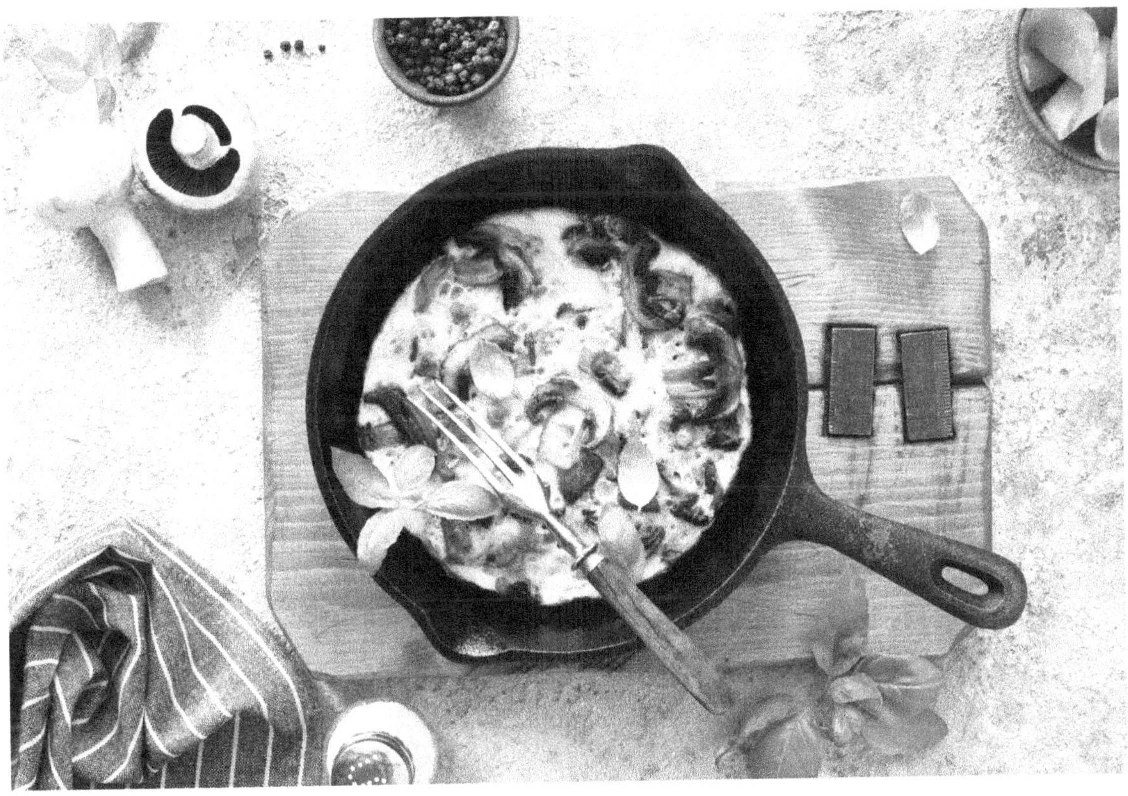

A healthy breakfast is the first step in a day that brings your brain power back to full capacity and can help you be more productive throughout the day. A ham and mushroom omelet breakfast with boiled eggs, seasoned with salt, pepper, nutmeg, cayenne pepper, dried thyme leaves or oregano leaves (chop before use), dried parsley leaves, or dry basil leaves is the best breakfast.

Serving size: 1

Cooking time: 6 minutes

Ingredients:

- 2 tbsp. ghee
- ¼ cup coconut milk
- 3 eggs
- 4 oz. smoked ham; chopped
- 3 oz. mushrooms; sliced
- 1 cup arugula; torn
- A pinch of black pepper

Instructions:

Heat a pan with half of the ghee over medium heat, add mushrooms, stir and cook for 3 minutes.

Add ham, stir; cook for 2-3 minutes more and transfer everything to a plate.

In a bowl, mix eggs with coconut milk and black pepper and whisk well.

Heat the pan with the rest of the ghee over medium heat, add eggs, spread into the pan, cook for a couple of minutes, start stirring and cook until eggs are completely done.

Transfer this to a serving bowl; add mushrooms mix on top and arugula. Toss everything to coat well and serve right away.

Chapter 2: Meat and Chicken recipes

Beef Soup

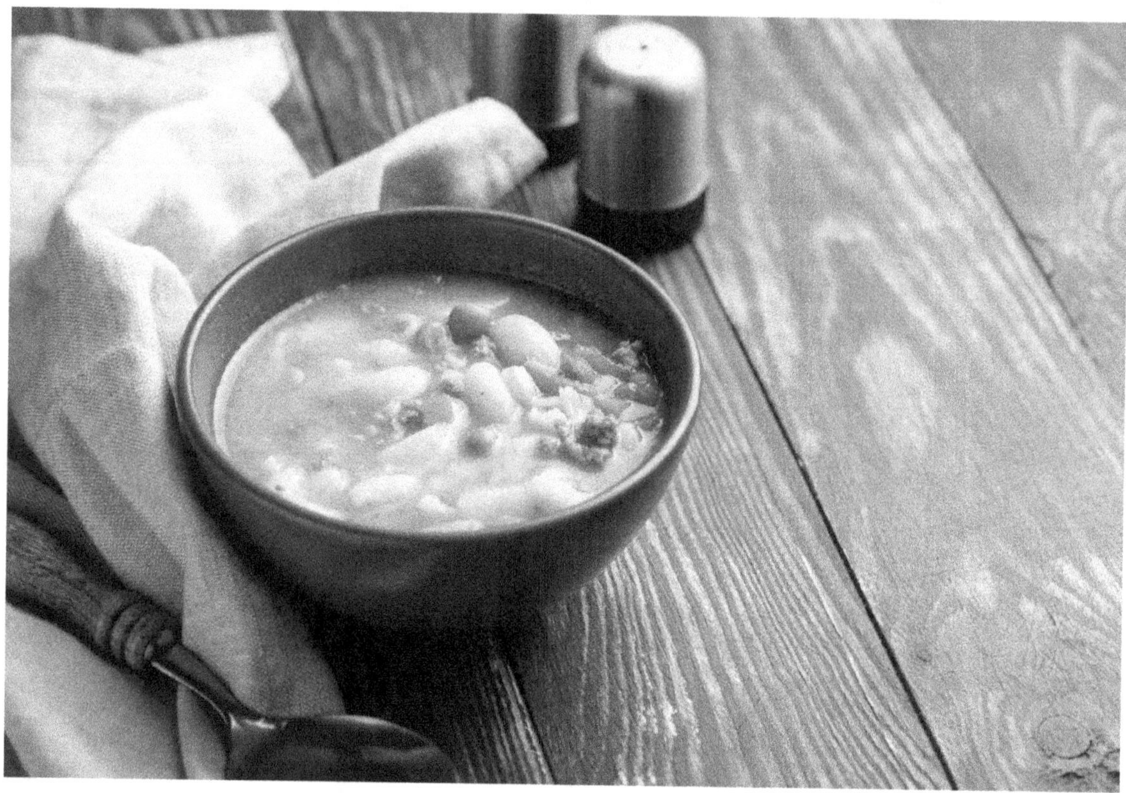

Beef soup is a savory broth made with beef and vegetables. The dish can be served either as a stew or as an individual course on its own. Some people like their soup thicker than others who prefer it thinner, while some like it spicy while others prefer mild flavors.

Serving size: 6

Cooking time: 1 hour

Ingredients:

- 1 lb. beef, ground
- 1 lb. sausage, sliced
- 4 cups beef stock
- 30 oz. canned tomatoes, diced
- 1 green bell pepper, chopped
- 3 zucchinis, chopped
- 1 cup celery, chopped
- 1 tsp. Italian seasoning
- ½ yellow onion, chopped
- ½ teaspoon oregano, dried
- ½ teaspoon basil, dried
- ¼ teaspoon garlic powder
- Salt and black pepper to the taste

Instructions:

Cook until it browns and drains excess fat.

Add tomatoes, zucchini, bell pepper, celery, onion, Italian seasoning, basil, oregano, garlic powder, salt, pepper to the taste and the stock, stir and boil, reducing heat medium-low, and simmer for 1 hour.

Pulled Pork

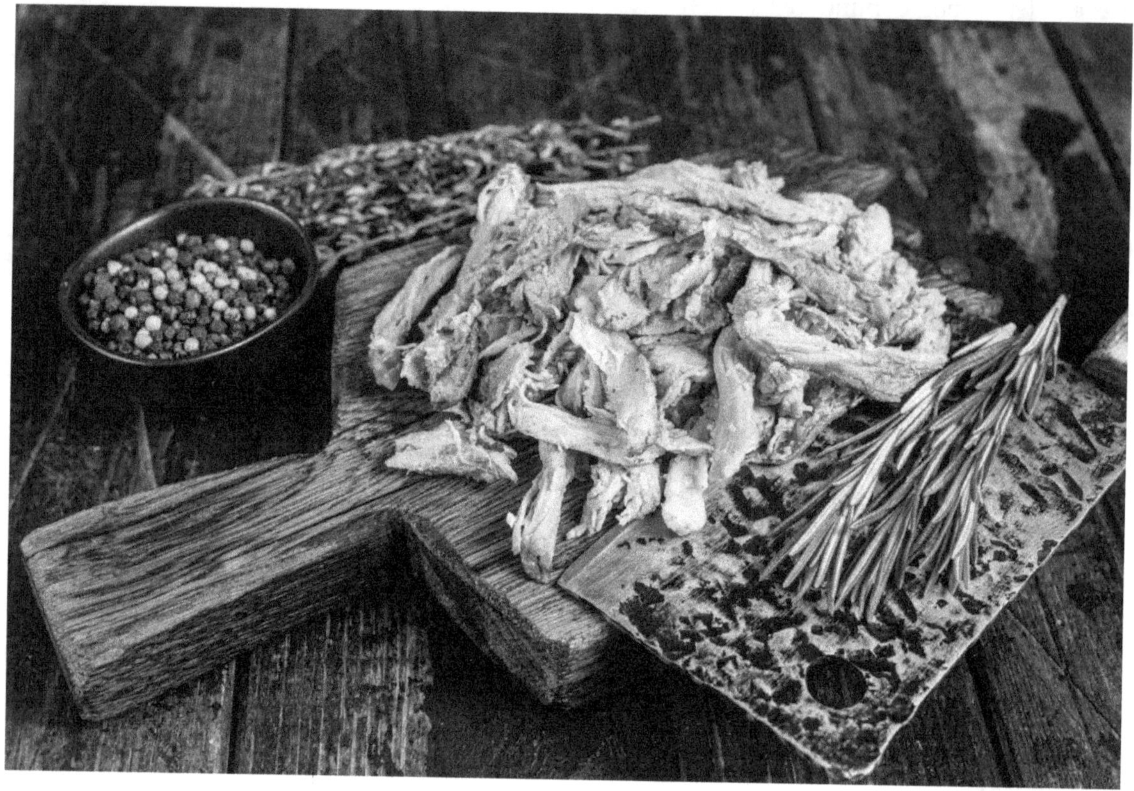

Serving size: 4

Cooking time: 8 hours 28 minutes

Ingredients:

- ½ cup salsa
- ½ cup beef stock
- ½ cup enchilada sauce
- 3 lbs. organic pork shoulder
- 2 green chilies; chopped
- 1 tbsp. garlic powder
- 1 tbsp. chili powder
- 1 tsp. onion powder
- 1 tsp. cumin
- 1 tsp. paprika
- Black pepper to the taste

Instructions:

In a bowl, mix chili powder with onion and garlic one.

Add cumin, paprika, and pepper to the taste and stir everything.

Add pork, rub well, and keep in the fridge for 12 hours.

Transfer pork to your slow cooker, add enchilada sauce, stock, salsa and green chilies, stir; cover and cook on Low for 8 hours.

Transfer pork to a plate, leave aside to cool down, and shred.

Strain sauce from slow cooker into a pan, bring to a boil over medium heat and simmer for 8 minutes stirring all the time.

Add shredded pork to the sauce, stir; reduce heat to medium and cook for 20 more minutes. Divide between plates and serve hot.

Grilled Lamb Chops

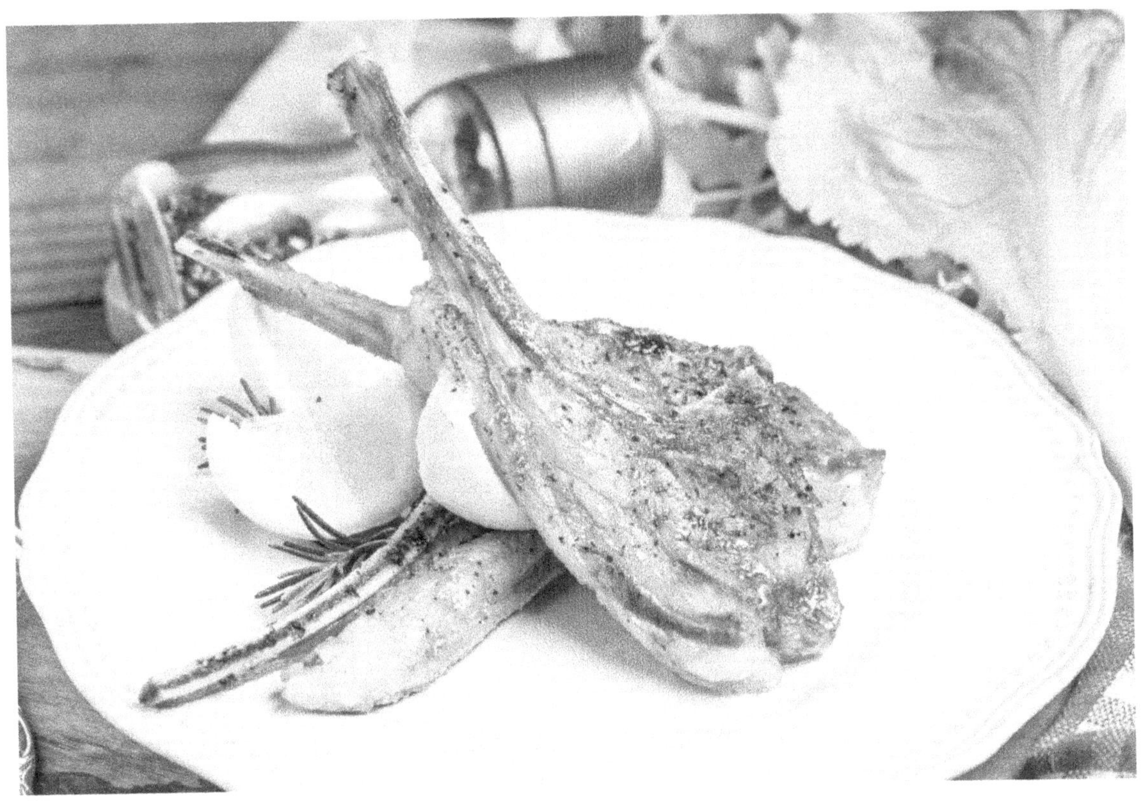

A good cut of lamb is delicious. The meat has a rich flavor and meaty texture that any other animal can't replicate. The meat is flavorful, juicy, and tender while cooking.

Grilled lamb chops are the perfect addition to a summer evening meal. They're great with a side of couscous and vegetables for flavor and texture.

Serving size: 6

Cooking time: 4 minutes

Ingredients:

- 3 tbsp. coconut amino
- 4 tbsp. extra virgin olive oil
- 8 lamb chops
- A pinch of sea salt
- Black pepper to the taste
- 2 garlic cloves; minced
- 2 tbsp. ginger; minced
- 1 tbsp. parsley leaves; chopped

Instructions:

In a bowl, mix olive oil with coconut amino, garlic, ginger, and parsley and stir well.

Season lamb chops with a pinch of sea salt and pepper to the taste, place the chops on the grill (medium-high heat), and cook for 4 minutes per side, basting all the time with the marinade you've made.

Divide lamb chops on plates, leave aside to cool down for 4 minutes, and serve.

Lamb Chops and Mint Sauce

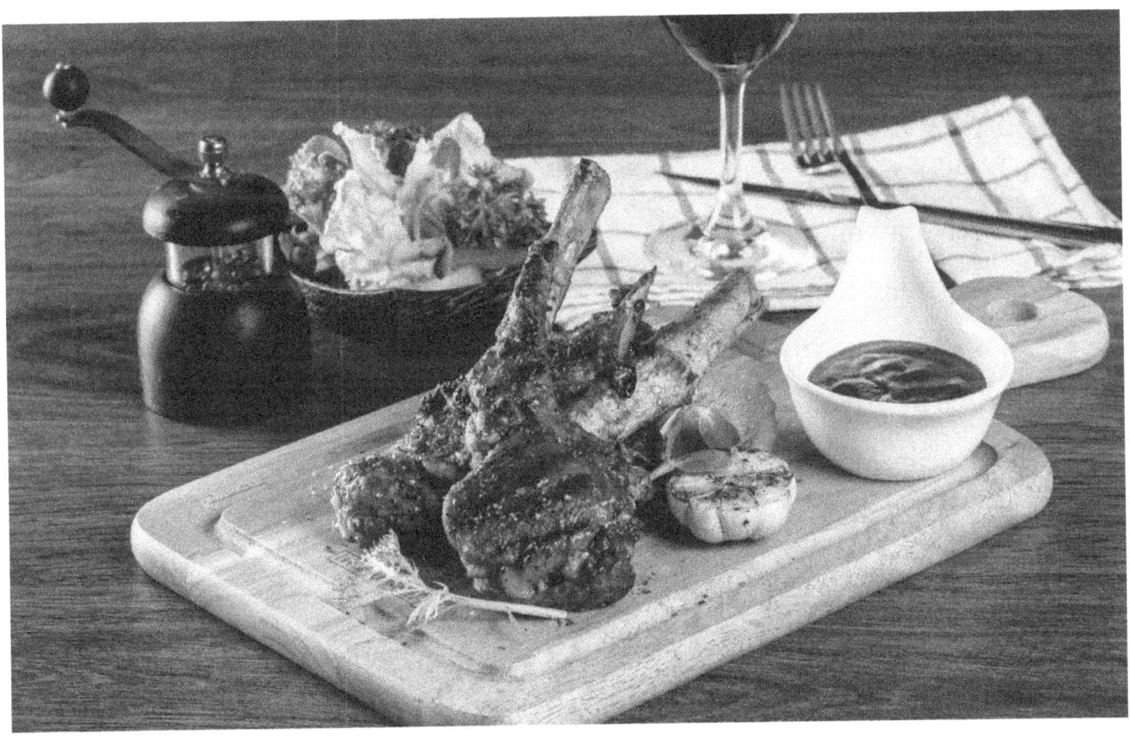

Both lamb and mint sauce make an excellent pairing for any Sunday night meal. You can jazz up the mint sauce with several fresh ingredients, including dill, thyme, or different types of wine or vinegar. This recipe relies on the classic parsley-shallot combination to lend a bright note to the savory lamb chops.

Serving size: 4

Cooking time: 5 minutes

Ingredients:

- 2 garlic cloves; minced
- 1 tbsp. lemon zest
- 1 tbsp. oregano; chopped
- 8 lamb chops
- 2/3 cup olive oil
- 1/3 cup mint; chopped
- 2 tbsp. balsamic vinegar
- A pinch of sea salt
- Black pepper to the taste
- 3 tbsp. Dijon mustard

Instructions:

In a bowl mix, oil with oregano, garlic, and lemon zest and whisk well.

Brush lamb chops with this mix, season them with a pinch of salt and black pepper to the taste, place the chops on the grill (medium-high heat), and cook for 5 minutes on each side.

In a bowl, mix mustard with a pinch of salt, mint, vinegar, and black pepper and whisk well.

Divide lamb chops on plates, drizzle mint sauce over them, and serve.

Beef Tenderloin with Special Sauce

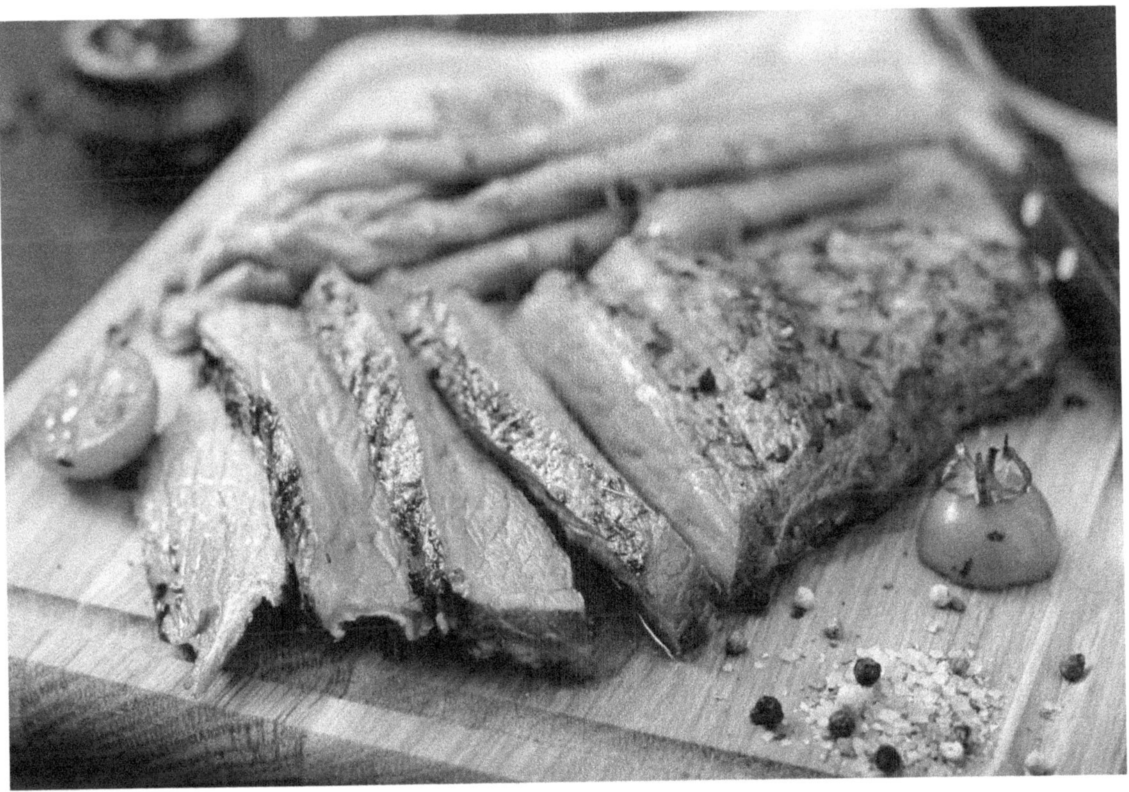

This is a recipe for very delicious and succulent beef tenderloin. You will need minced garlic, soy sauce, sherry, balsamic vinegar, Worcestershire sauce, sesame oil, and cornstarch. It's also recommended to use the beef filet in this recipe because it's tenderer than flank steak if you have time to marinate your filet overnight in its juices before cooking it, that would be best.

Serving size: 4

Cooking time: 27 minutes

Ingredients:

- 3 tbsp. Dijon mustard
- 3 lbs. beef tenderloin
- A pinch of sea salt
- Black pepper to the taste
- 1 tbsp. coconut oil
- 3 tbsp. balsamic vinegar

For the sauce:

- 3 tbsp. basil leaves; chopped
- ½ cup parsley leaves; chopped
- Zest from 1 lemon
- 2 garlic cloves; finely chopped
- A pinch of sea salt
- Black pepper to the taste
- ¼ cup extra virgin olive oil

Instructions:

In a bowl mix, mustard with vinegar, stir very well, and leave aside.

Season beef with a pinch of sea salt and pepper to the taste, put in a pan heated with the coconut oil over medium-high, heat and cook for 2 minutes on each side.

Transfer beef to a baking pan, cover with the mustard mix, introduce in the oven at 475°F and bake for 25 minutes.

Meanwhile, in a bowl, mix parsley with basil, lemon zest, garlic, olive oil, a pinch of sea salt and pepper to the taste and whisk very well.

Take beef tenderloin out of the oven, leave aside for a few minutes to cool down, slice, and divide between plates. Serve with herbs sauce on the side.

Pork Tenderloin with Carrot Puree

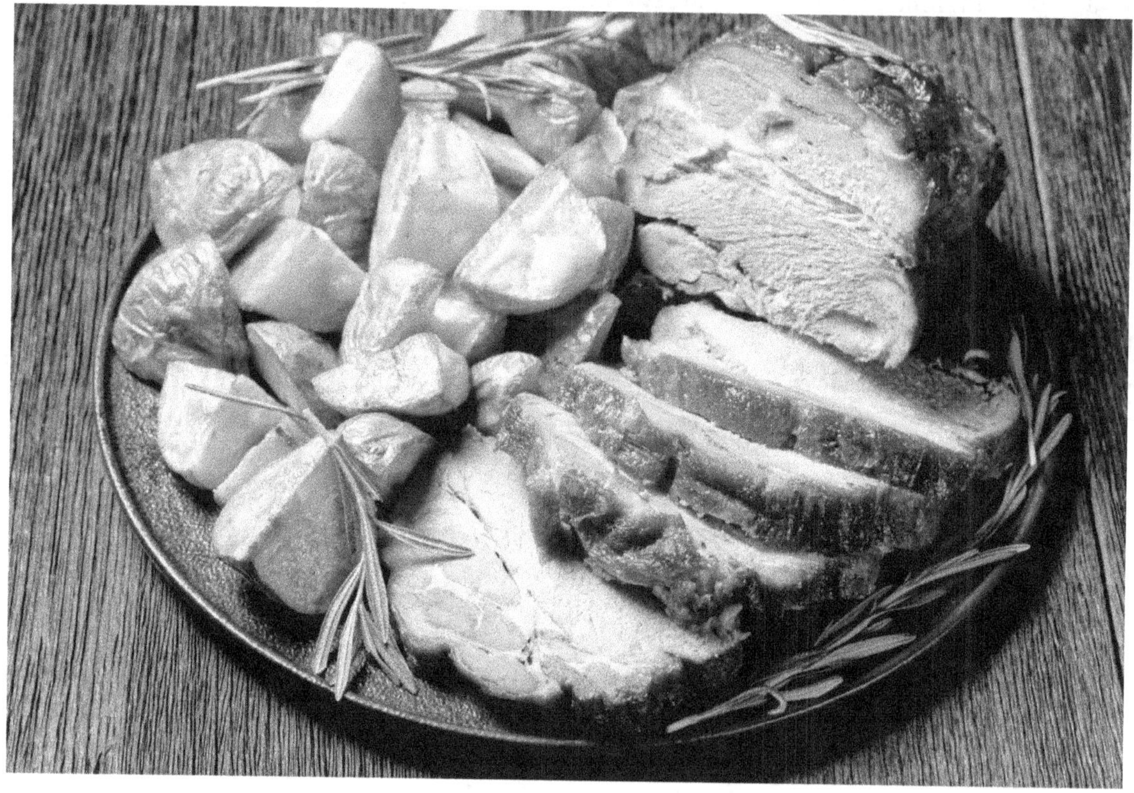

This recipe combines the natural sweetness of carrots with savory spices, yielding a delicious dish perfect for any occasion.

Serving size: 4

Cooking time: 1 hour

Ingredients:

- 2 sausages; casings removed
- A handful arugula
- Black pepper to the taste
- 1 grass-fed pork tenderloin
- 1 tbsp. coconut oil

For the puree:

- 1 sweet potato; chopped
- 3 carrots; chopped
- A pinch of sea salt
- Black pepper to the taste
- 1 tbsp. curry paste

For the sauce:

- 2 tbsp. balsamic vinegar
- 1 tsp. mustard
- 2 shallots; finely chopped
- Black pepper to the taste
- 4 tbsp. extra virgin olive oil

Instructions:

Slice pork tenderloin in half horizontally but not all the way and open it up.

Use a meat tenderizer to even it up.

Place sausage in the middle, roll pork around it, tie with twine, season pepper to the taste and leave aside.

Heat an oven-proof pan with the coconut oil over medium-high heat, add pork roll, cook for 3 minutes on each side, introduce in the oven at 350°F and bake for 25 minutes.

Meanwhile, put potatoes and carrots in a pot, add water to cover, bring to a boil over medium-high heat, cook for 20 minutes, drain and transfer to your food processor.

Pulse a few times until you obtain a puree, add a pinch of sea salt and pepper to the taste, blend again, transfer to a bowl and leave aside.

Take pork roll out of the oven, slice and divide between plates.

Heat a pan with the olive oil over medium-high heat, add shallots, stir and cook for 10 minutes.

Add balsamic vinegar, mustard, pepper, stir well and take off the heat. Divide carrots puree next to pork slices, drizzle vinegar sauce and serve with arugula on the side.

Beef and Wonderful Gravy

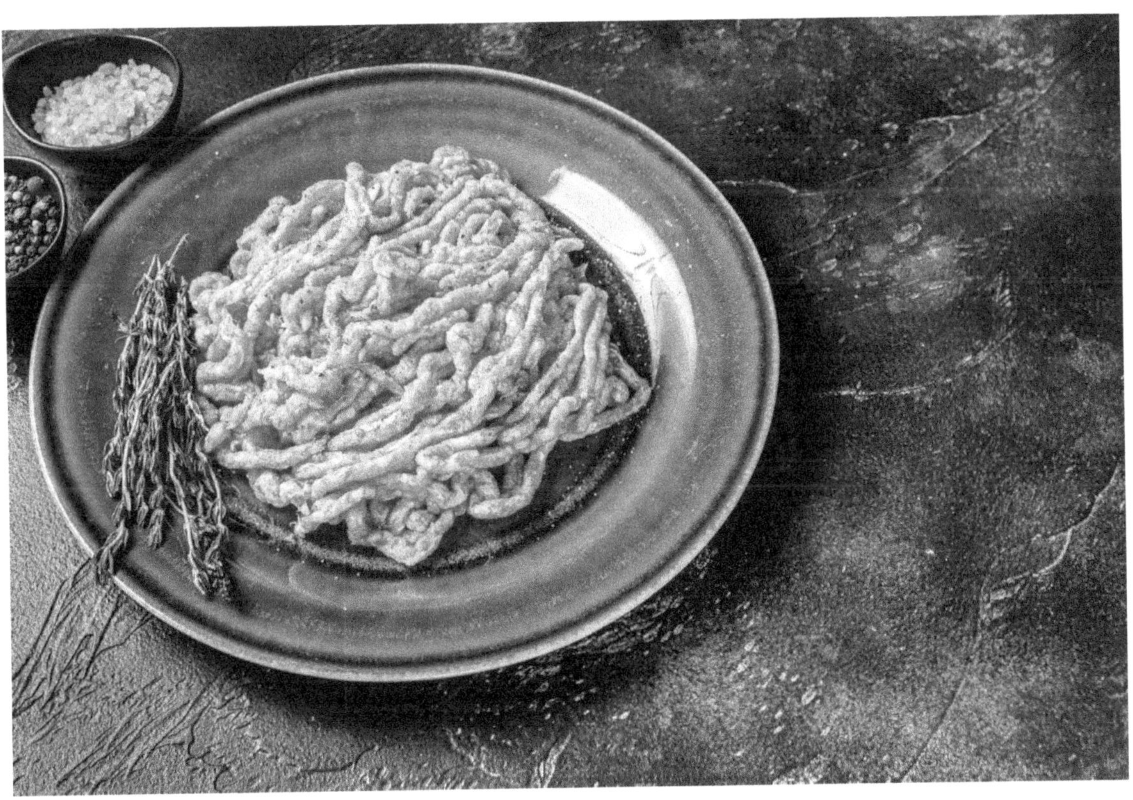

If you're looking for a way to jazz up your homemade meatloaf, this is it. It's a simple recipe but tasty, with just the right amount of heat from the pepper flakes and chili powder. Just make sure to start here on top of your loaf before adding any more ingredients.

Serving size: 4

Cooking time: 7 minutes

Ingredients:

- 1 egg; whisked
- 1 tbsp. mustard
- 1 tbsp. tomato paste
- 1 tsp. garlic powder
- 1 tsp. onion powder
- Some coconut oil for cooking
- A pinch of sea salt and black pepper to the taste
- 1½ lb. beef; ground

For the gravy:

- 2 tsp. parsley; chopped
- 2 tbsp. ghee
- 1 tsp. tapioca
- 1 small yellow onion; chopped
- 1¼ cups beef stock
- Black pepper to the taste

Instructions:

In a bowl mix, beef with tomato paste, egg, mustard, onion powder, garlic powder, a pinch of salt, and black pepper to the taste and stir well.

Heat a pan with the ghee over medium heat, add onion, stir and cook for 2 minutes.

Add stock, some black pepper, tapioca mixed with water. Stir; cook until it thickens and take off the heat.

Shape 4 patties from the beef mix. Heat up a pan with the coconut oil over medium-high heat, add beef patties and cook for 5 minutes on each side.

Pour the gravy over beef patties, sprinkle parsley on top, cook for a couple more minutes, divide between plates and serve.

Lamb And Eggplant Puree

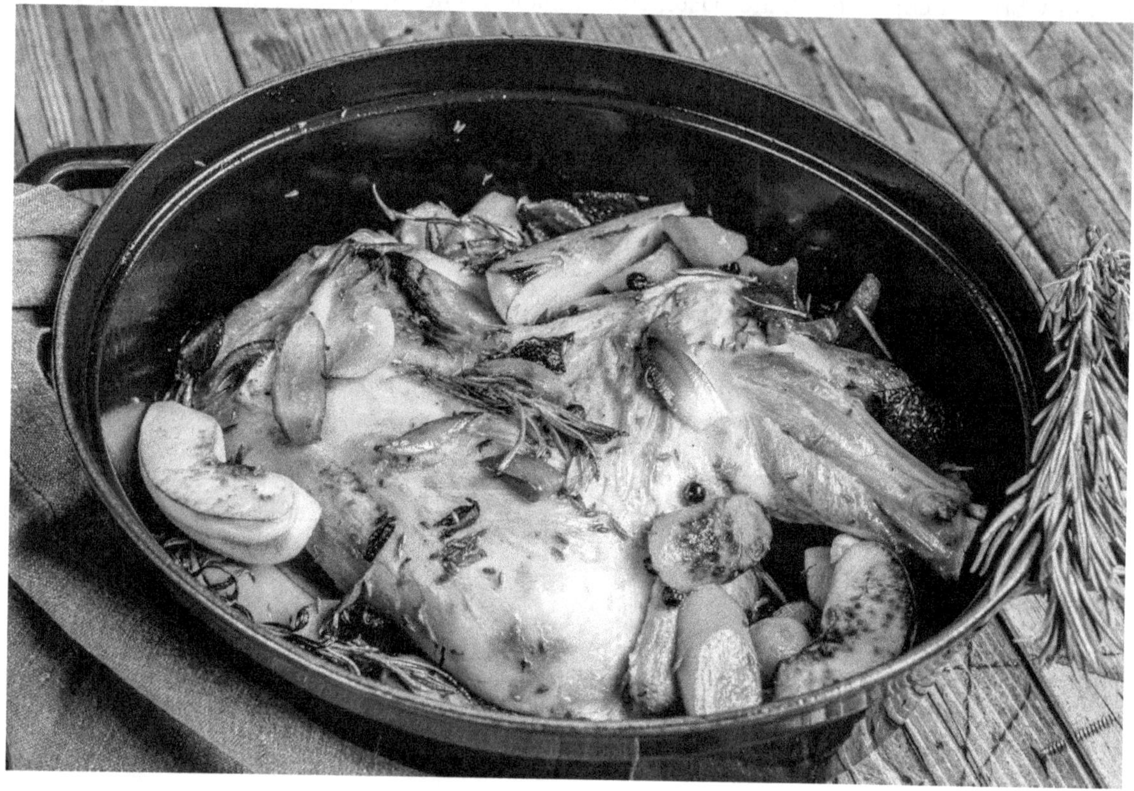

A traditional Lebanese dish with Mediterranean roots, lamb, and eggplant puree is a hearty and satisfying dish. It's made with ground lamb, onions, garlic, thyme leaves, fresh tomatoes, or canned tomatoes when in season and white wine.

Serving size: 4

Cooking time: 2 hours 55 minutes

Ingredients:

- 4 lamb shoulder chops
- 1 tbsp. ghee
- A pinch of sea salt
- Black pepper to the taste
- 1 cup yellow onion; chopped
- 7 oz. tomato paste
- 2 garlic cloves; minced
- 3 cups water
- 8 oz. white mushrooms; halved

For the eggplant puree:

- Juice of 1 lemon
- ¼ tsp. white pepper
- 2 eggplants
- 4 tbsp. ghee
- A pinch of sea salt

Instructions:

Place eggplants on your preheated grill, cook for 30 minutes, flipping them from time to time, leave them to cool down and peel.

In your food processor, mix eggplant flesh with a pinch of salt, white pepper, lemon juice and 4 tbsp. ghee and pulse really well.

Spoon eggplant puree on plates and leave aside for now.

Heat a pot with 1 tbsp. ghee, add lamb chops, season with a pinch of salt and black pepper to the taste, stir; brown them for a few minutes on each side and transfer to a plate.

Heat the pot again over medium-high heat, add onion, stir and cook for a couple of minutes.

Add garlic, stir and cook for 1 minute more.

Add mushrooms and tomato paste, stir and cook for 3 minutes more.

Add water, return lamb chops, stir; bring to a simmer, cover pot, reduce heat to medium-low heat and cook everything for 2 hours and 20 minutes. Divide lamb chops on eggplant puree and serve.

Rosemary Citrus Chicken

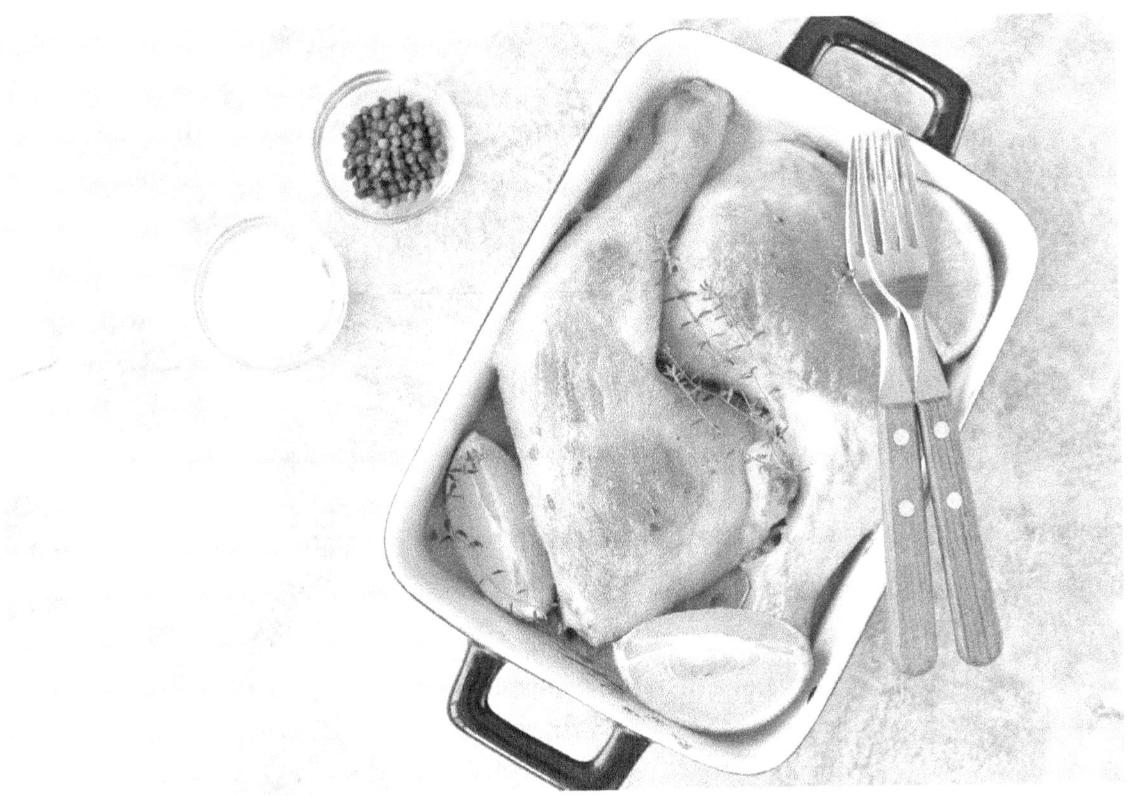

This oven-cooked citrus marinade is so easy to make! All you need is some chicken, some rosemary, and a few lemons. This recipe is perfect for those looking to incorporate more fresh herbs into their diet. Rosemary is a flavorful herb that pairs well with citrus flavors, making it the perfect addition to this healthy chicken dish!

Serving size: 3

Cooking time: 8 hours

Ingredients:

- 4 fresh rosemary sprigs
- 4 orange slices
- 1 tablespoon honey
- 2 tablespoons freshly-squeezed orange juice
- 3 tablespoons lemon juice
- 1 pound chicken breast (boneless and skinless)
- Salt and pepper to taste

Instructions:

Generously rub all sides of chicken breasts with salt and pepper and put them in a slow cooker.

Whisk honey, orange juice, and lemon juice in a bowl until combined. Pour over the meat in the slow cooker. Add the rosemary and orange slices on top of the meat.

Cover the slow cooker and cook for 8 hours on a low-temperature setting.

Turkey Casserole

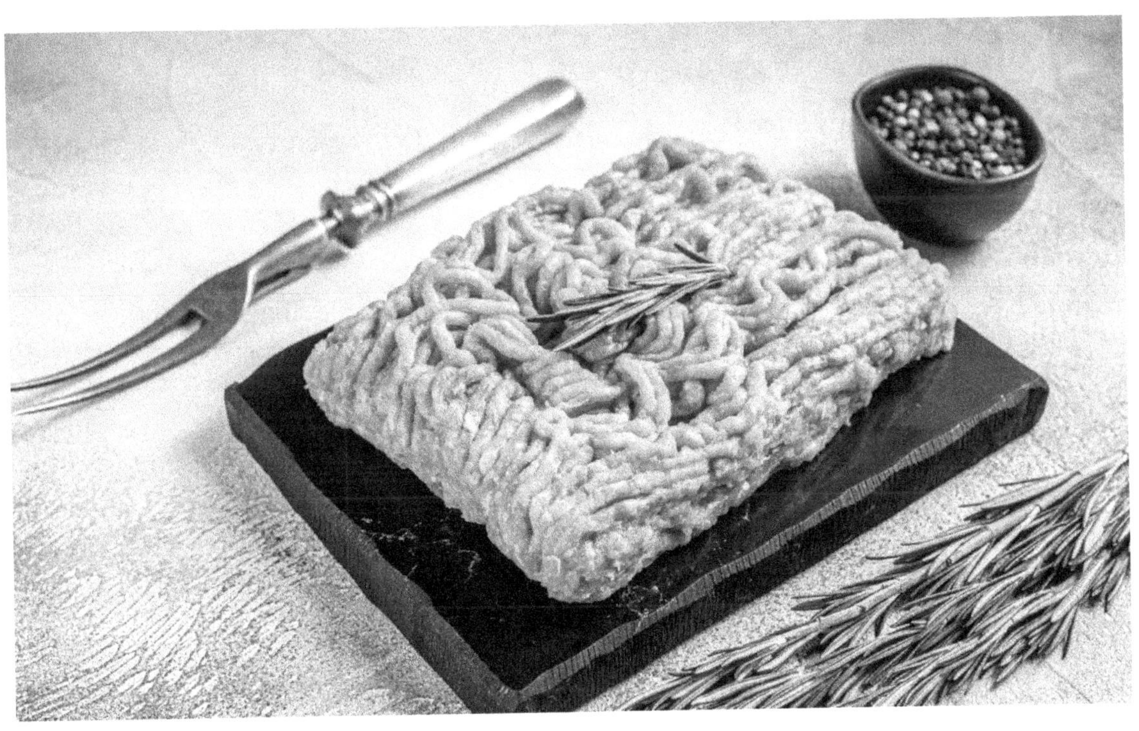

Most people love turkey, and who can blame them? The only thing better than a juicy, melt-in-your-mouth turkey is a rich, savory casserole made with a said bird!

This dish is a fitting tribute to the glorious bird and its feathers. It is made with turkey, potatoes, eggs, cornbread topping, and more.

Serving size: 6

Cooking time: 1 hour 17 minutes

Ingredients:

- 1 sweet potato; chopped

- 1 lb. turkey meat; ground

- 1 eggplant; thinly sliced

- 1 yellow onion; finely chopped

- 1 tbsp. garlic; finely minced

- A pinch of sea salt

- Black pepper to the taste

- ¼ tsp. chili powder

- ¼ tsp. cumin

- 15 oz. canned tomatoes; chopped and drained

- 8 oz. tomato paste

- A drizzle of olive oil

- ½ tsp. tarragon flakes

- 1/8 tsp. cardamom; ground

- 1/8 tsp. oregano

For the sauce:

- 1 tbsp. almond flour

- 1 cup almond milk

- 1½ tbsp. extra virgin olive oil

- 1 tbsp. coconut flour

Instructions:

Heat a pan over medium-high heat, add turkey meat, onion, and garlic, stir and cook until the meat turns brown.

Add tomatoes, tomato paste, and sweet potatoes, stir and cook for 5 minutes.

Add a pinch of sea salt, pepper to the taste, chili powder, cumin, oregano, tarragon flakes, and cardamom, stir well, and cook for 2 minutes.

Grease a baking dish with a drizzle of olive oil, arrange eggplant slices on the bottom and add turkey mixture on top.

Spread turkey mix evenly, introduce dish in the oven at 350°F and bake for 15 minutes.

Meanwhile, heat a pot over medium-high heat, add the rest of the olive oil, almond flour, and coconut one, stir well 1 minute, reduce heat, add almond milk and stir well.

Cook this for 10 minutes.

Take the baking dish out of the oven and pour this almond milk mixture over it.

Introduce in the oven again and bake for 45 minutes. Take the casserole out of the oven, leave aside a few minutes to cool down, slice and divide between plates and serve.

Chicken Thighs with Tasty Squash

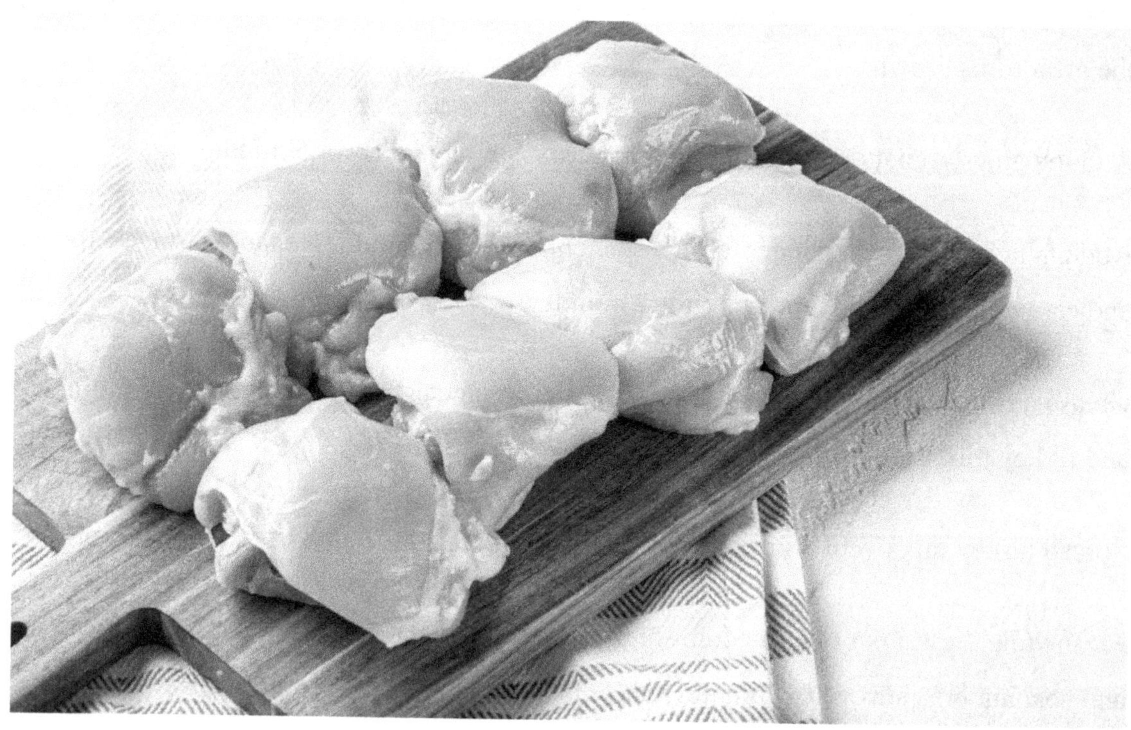

Whether you're roasting, grilling, or frying, these chicken thighs will be a hit with everyone. The savory sauce is made with four ingredients, and it's so simple. This dish is perfect for a weeknight dinner because it practically cooks itself in the oven! It comes out juicy and tender every time, no matter what cooking method you use.

Serving size: 6

Cooking time: 25 minutes

Ingredients:

- 6 chicken thighs; boneless and skinless
- ½ lb. bacon; chopped
- 2 tbsp. coconut oil
- A pinch of sea salt
- A handful sage; chopped
- Black pepper to the taste
- 3 cups butternut squash; cubed

Instructions:

Heat a pan over medium heat, add bacon, cook until it's crispy, drain on paper towels, transfer to a plate, crumble and leave aside for now.

Heat the same pan over medium heat, add butternut squash, a pinch of salt and black pepper to the taste, stir; cook until it's soft, transfer to a plate, and also leave aside.

Heat the pan again with the coconut oil over medium-high heat, add chicken, salt, and pepper and cook for 10 minutes, turning often.

Take the pan off the heat, add squash, introduce in the oven at 425°F and bake for 15 minutes. Divide chicken and butternut on plates, top with sage and bacon, and serve.

Chicken Meatballs

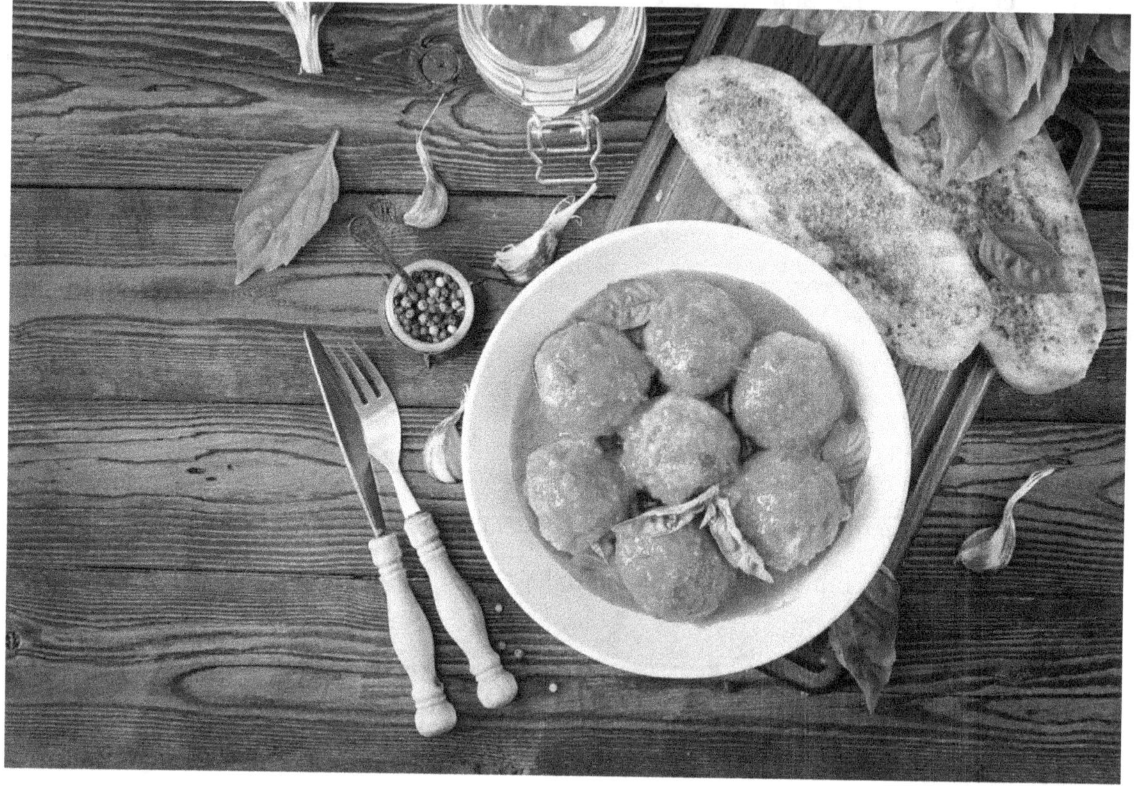

In this recipe, we make ground chicken meatballs that are cooked in a lemon-mushroom sauce. You'll need a fair amount of fat on hand to cook these properly, but they are worth the extra effort. Your family and friends will be amazed when you reveal your culinary secrets!

This is one of those recipes that gets better with time.

Serving size: 4

Cooking time: 30 minutes

Ingredients:

- 1 tsp. sweet paprika
- 1 pineapple; diced
- 1 egg
- 2 lbs. chicken meat; ground
- A pinch of sea salt
- Black pepper to the taste
- 1 tsp. garlic powder
- 1 tsp. onion powder

For the sauce:

- ¼ cup coconut amino
- 4 tbsp. ketchup
- 1 tbsp. ginger; grated
- ½ cup pineapple juice
- 2 tsp. raw honey
- ½ tsp. red pepper flakes
- Salt and black pepper to the taste
- 1 tbsp. garlic; minced

Instructions:

In a pot, mix amino with ketchup, ginger, pineapple sauce, garlic, pepper flakes, honey, a pinch of sea salt and pepper to the taste, stir well, bring to a boil over medium heat, simmer for 8 minutes and take off the heat.

In a bowl, mix chicken meat with paprika, egg, onion powder, garlic powder, salt, and black pepper to the taste and stir well.

Shape meatballs, arrange them on a lined baking sheet, introduce them in the oven at 475°F and bake for 15 minutes.

Heat a pan over medium heat, add pineapple pieces, stir and cook for 2 minutes.

Add baked meatballs, pour sauce you've made at the beginning, stir gently, cook for 5 minutes, divide between plates and serve.

Beef and Cabbage Delight

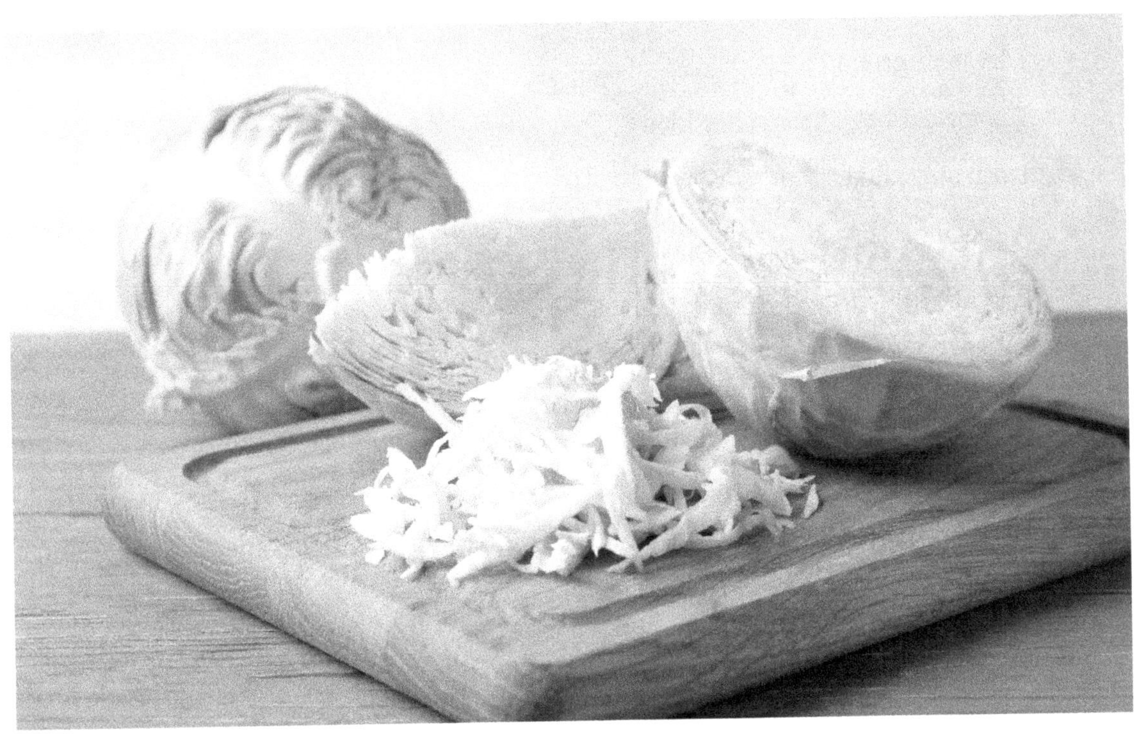

What is your favorite food? A national dish would be a great answer, but if you're looking for something easy to make with ingredients sitting in the cupboard, then try this one - it's like a stir-fry meets cabbage soup.

This meal is filling and tastes good hot or cold, so it's perfect when you want something on the go.

Serving time: 4

Cooking time: 10 minutes

Ingredients:

- 1 onion chopped
- 1 lb. beef ground
- 1 Napa cabbage head, shredded
- 1 carrot, grated
- A pinch of sea salt
- Black pepper to the taste
- 2 tbsp. coconut oil

Instructions:

Heat a pan with the oil over medium-high heat, add onion and beef, stir and brown them for 5 minutes.

Add carrots, cabbage, a pinch of salt and black pepper to the taste, stir and cook for 5 minutes more. Divide between plates and serve.

Chapter 3: Seafood recipes

Shrimp and Cauliflower Rice

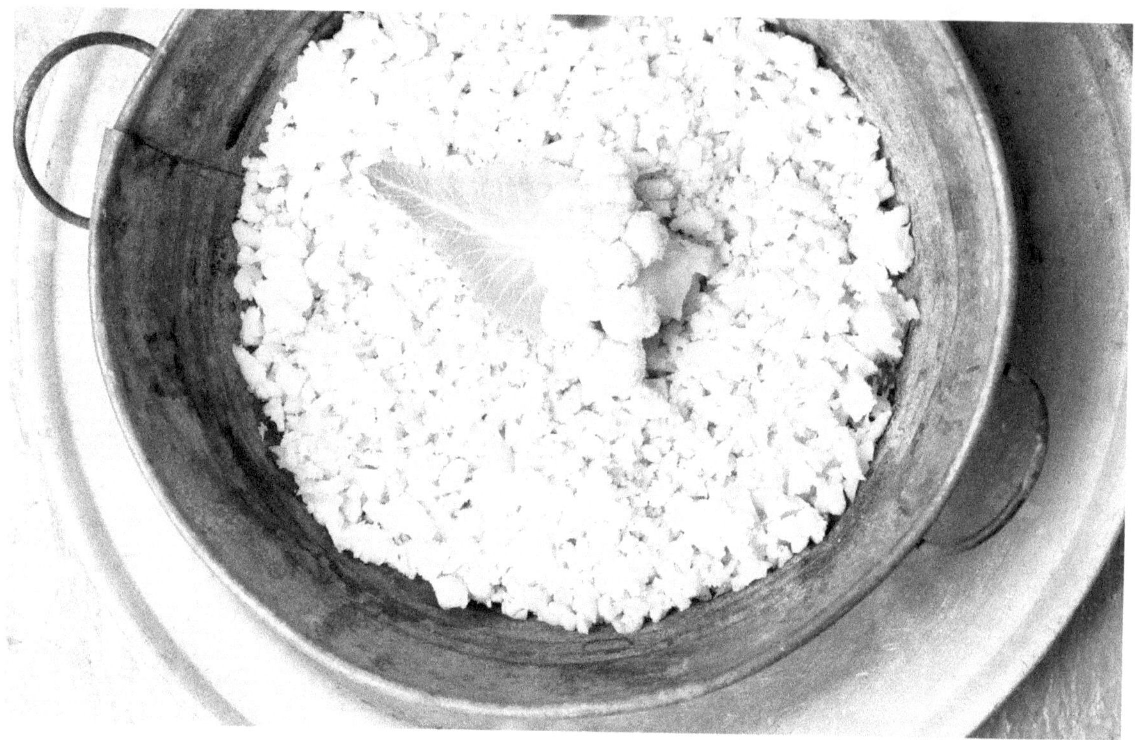

Shrimp and Cauliflower Rice is a healthier alternative to traditional rice dishes. With 45 calories for the entire meal, it's lower in fat and higher in fiber than rice, making it a perfect dish for on the go or when you're watching your waistline.

Serving size: 4

Cooking time: 10 minutes

Ingredients:

- 1 tbsp. ghee
- 1 cauliflower head; florets separated
- ¼ cup coconut milk
- 1 lb. shrimp; peeled and deveined
- 2 garlic cloves; minced
- 8 oz. mushrooms; sliced
- 4 bacon slices
- A pinch of red pepper flakes
- A handful mixed parsley and chives; chopped
- ½ cup beef stock
- Black pepper to the taste

Instructions:

Heat a pan over medium-high heat, add bacon slices, cook until crispy, drain grease on paper towels, and leave them aside for now.

Put cauliflower florets in your food processor, blend until you obtain your "rice," and transfer to a heated pan over medium-high heat.

Cook cauliflower rice for 5 minutes, stirring often.

Add coconut milk and 1 tbsp. ghee, stir, and cook for a couple more minutes.

Blend everything using an immersion blender, add black pepper to the taste, stir, reduce heat to low and continue cooking for a few minutes more.

Heat the pan where you cooked the bacon over medium-high heat, add shrimp, cook for 2 minutes on each side and transfer them to a plate.

Heat the pan again, add mushrooms, stir and cook for a few minutes as well.

Add garlic, pepper flakes, and some black pepper, stir and cook for 1 minute. Add stock, return shrimp to pan, stir and cook until stock evaporates.

Divide cauliflower rice on plates, top with shrimp and mushrooms mix, top with crispy bacon, and sprinkle parsley and chives.

Glazed Salmon

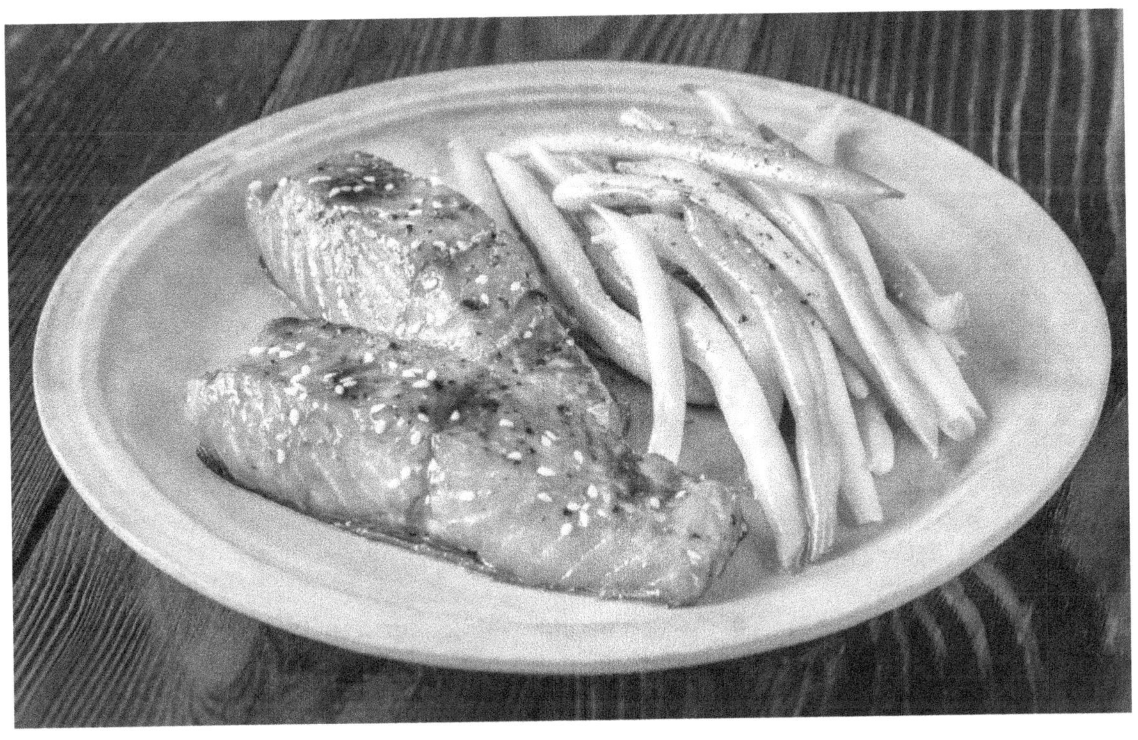

You will find that glazed salmon is not only easy to prepare, but it also has a delightful taste. This dish perfectly combines some unusual flavors!

Serving size: 4

Cooking time: 15 minutes

Ingredients:

- 2 tbsp. pure maple syrup
- 4 salmon fillets, skin-on
- Salt and white pepper to taste
- 2 tsp. Dijon mustard
- Juice and zest from 1 orange
- 2 garlic cloves, finely chopped

Instructions:

In a bowl, mix maple syrup with orange zest, juice, mustard, salt, pepper, and garlic, and whisk well.

Arrange salmon in a baking dish, brush with the maple syrup and orange mix, introduce in the oven at 400°F and bake for 15 minutes.

Divide between plates and serve right away.

Lobster With Sauce

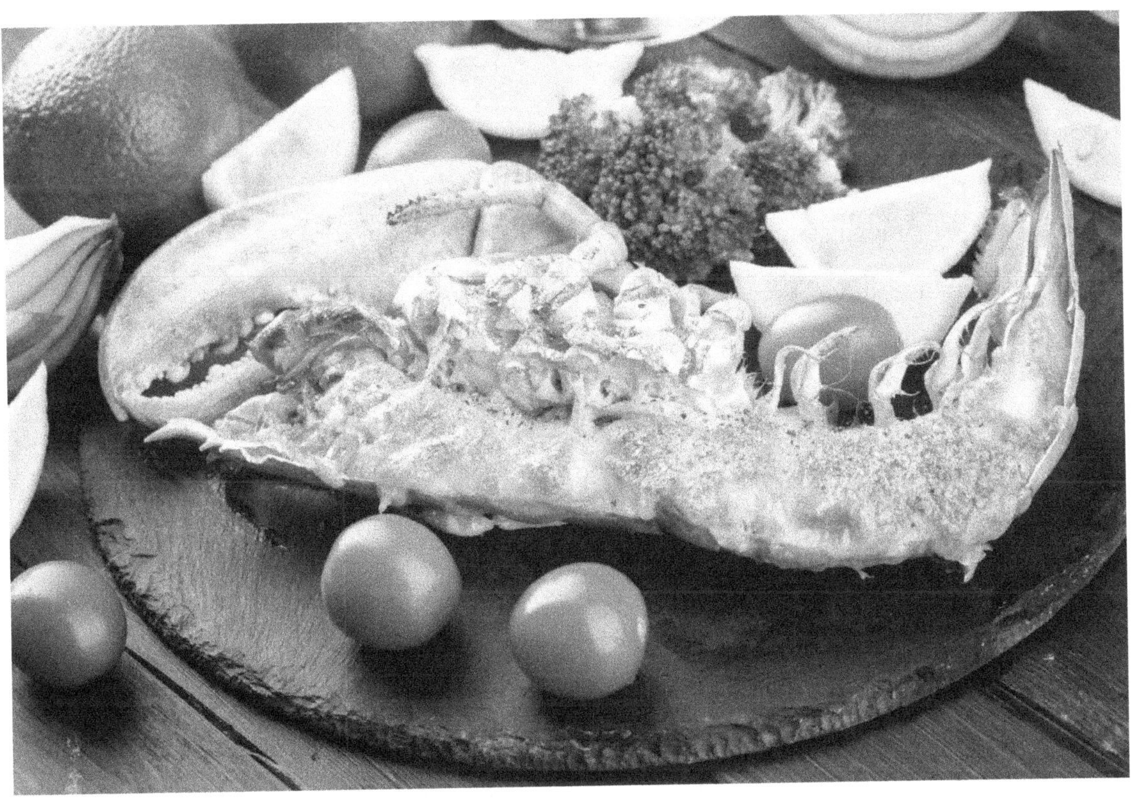

For those who don't have time for a long pasta to bake with vegetables and meat sauce, it's always good to have an alternative. This easy recipe is great for those of you looking for something quick and hearty. There is a simple creamy white wine sauce in between all the delicious lobster that takes just minutes to make. Once the sauce has thickened up, pour it over your pasta.

Serving size: 4

Cooking time: 7 minutes

Ingredients:

- ¼ cup ghee; melted
- 4 lobster tails
- A pinch of sea salt
- Black pepper to the taste
- 2 tbsp. Sriracha sauce
- 1 tbsp. lime juice
- 1 tbsp. chives; chopped
- Some parsley leaves; chopped for serving

Instructions:

In a bowl mix, Sriracha sauce with ghee, chives, a pinch of sea salt, pepper, and lime juice, and whisk well.

Cut lobster tails halfway through in the center, open with your fingers, fill them with half of the Sriracha mix, arrange on preheated grill over medium-high heat, cook for 4 minutes, flip and cook for 3 minutes more.

Divide lobster tails on plates, drizzle the rest of the Sriracha sauce, sprinkle parsley on top, and serve.

Scallops With Delicious Puree

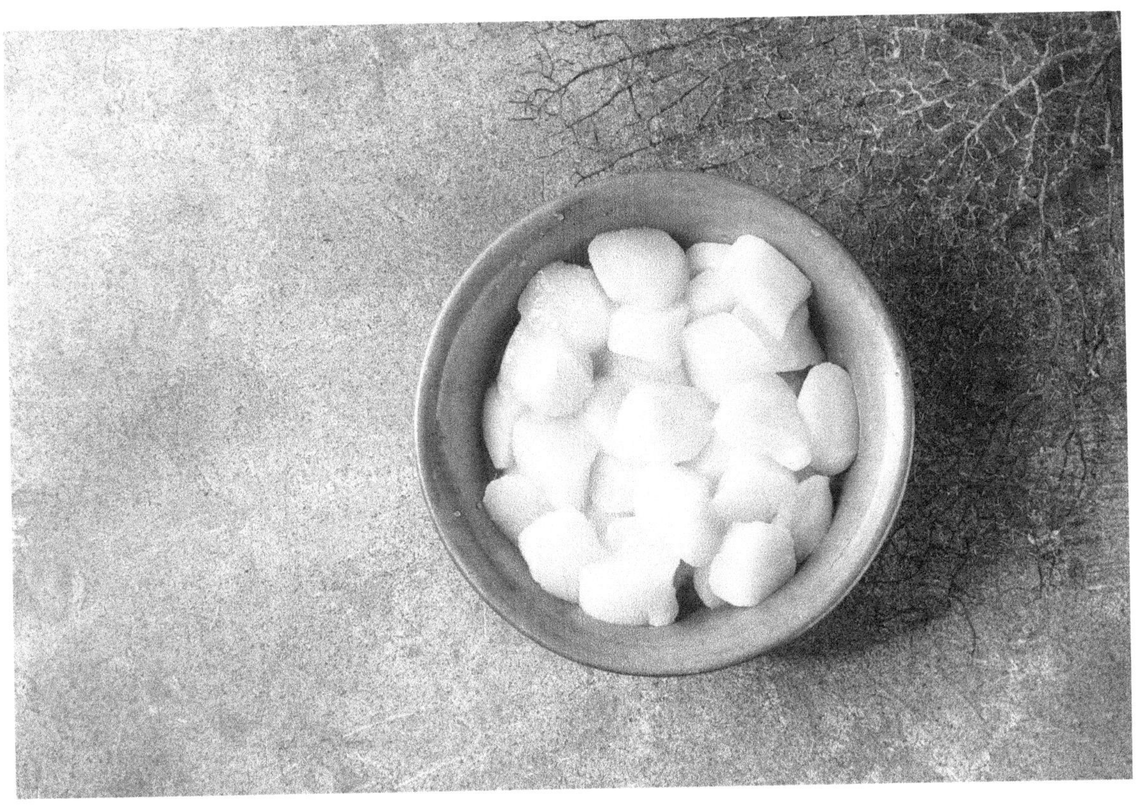

Yummy scallops with a delicious sauce served over a bed of fresh spinach and rice. It is a fantastic dish that is perfect for dinner. Plus, you can make it in under 20 minutes! To make everything taste even better, top it off with some wonderfully tangy balsamic vinegar to give the dish that special little something extra.

Serving size: 4

Cooking time: 3 minutes

Ingredients:

- 3 garlic cloves; minced
- 2 cups cauliflower florets; chopped
- 2 cups sweet potatoes; chopped
- 2 rosemary springs
- 12 sea scallops
- A pinch of sea salt
- Black pepper
- ¼ cup pine nuts; toasted
- 2 cups veggie stock
- 2 tbsp. extra virgin olive oil
- A handful chives; chopped

Instructions:

Put cauliflower, potatoes, and stock in a pot, bring to a boil over medium-high heat, reduce temperature and simmer until veggies are soft.

Drain veggies, transfer them to your blender, add a pinch of sea salt and pepper to the taste and pulse until you obtain a puree.

Heat a pan with the oil (medium-high), add rosemary and garlic, and cook for 1 minute.

Add scallops, cook them for 2 minutes, stirring, season them with pepper to the taste and take them off heat. Divide puree on small plates, arrange scallops on top, sprinkle chives and pine nuts at the end and serve.

Tuna And Chimichurri Sauce

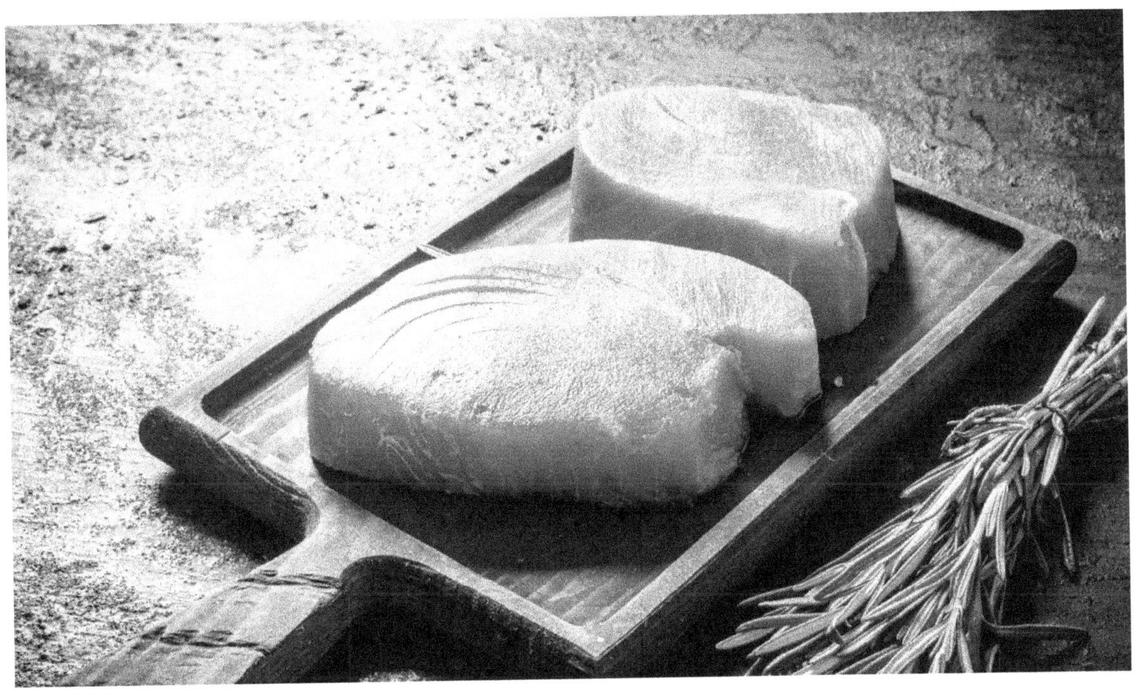

Tuna steaks are the perfect recipe for a satisfying meal. When they're seared in oil, they become nutty and crispy on the outside. Then you get to enjoy them with a delicious chimichurri sauce made from herbs, garlic, olive oil, and vinegar! This recipe is straightforward to prepare if you buy the pre-made chimichurri sauce at your local supermarket.

Serving size: 4

Cooking time: 2 minutes

Ingredients:

- 1 small red onion; chopped
- ½ cup cilantro; chopped
- 1/3 cup olive oil
- 2 tbsp. olive oil
- 1 jalapeno pepper; chopped
- 2 tbsp. basil; chopped
- 3 tbsp. vinegar
- 3 garlic cloves; minced
- 1 tsp. red pepper flakes
- 1 tsp. thyme; chopped
- A pinch of sea salt
- Black pepper to the taste
- 1 lb. sushi-grade tuna
- 2 avocados; pitted, peeled, and chopped
- 6 oz. arugula

Instructions:

In a bowl, mix 1/3 cup oil with onion, jalapeno, cilantro, basil, vinegar, garlic, parsley, pepper flakes, thyme, a pinch of salt, and black pepper and whisk well.

Heat up a pan with 2 tbsp. oil over medium-high heat, add tuna, season with a pinch of sea salt and black pepper, cook for 2 minutes on each side, transfer to a cutting board, leave aside to cool down and slice.

In a bowl mix, arugula with half of the chimichurri sauce you've made earlier, toss to coat well and divide between plates. Divide tuna slices, avocado pieces and drizzle the rest of the sauce on top.

Salmon With Avocado Sauce

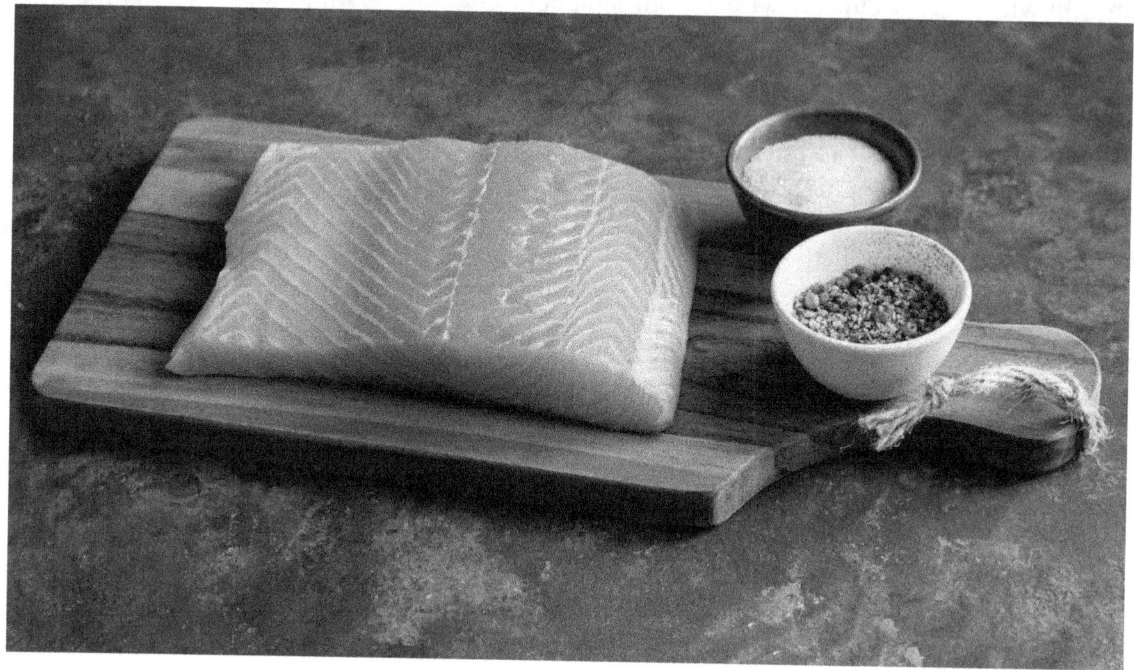

This savory dish will fill you up without making you feel sluggish or too full. It can be served with white rice, brown rice, or quinoa. Salmon is an excellent source of Omega-3s, and avocados are considered a "superfood" because they're so nutrient-dense!

Serving size: 5

Cooking time: 10 minutes

Ingredients:

- 1 tsp. cumin
- 1 tsp. sweet paprika
- 1 tsp. chili powder
- 1 tsp. onion powder
- ½ tsp. garlic powder
- 2 lbs. salmon filets; cut into 4 pieces
- A pinch of sea salt
- Black pepper to the taste

For the avocado sauce:

- 2 avocados; pitted, peeled and chopped
- 1 garlic clove; minced
- Juice from 1 lime
- 1 red onion; chopped
- 1 tbsp. extra virgin olive oil
- Black pepper to the taste
- 1 tbsp. cilantro; finely chopped

Instructions:

In a bowl mix, paprika with cumin, onion powder, garlic powder, chili powder, a pinch of sea salt, and pepper to the taste.

Add salmon pieces, toss to coat, and keep in the fridge for 20 minutes.

Put the avocado in a bowl and mash well with a fork.

Add red onion, garlic clove, lime juice, olive oil, chopped cilantro, and pepper to the taste and stir very well.

Take salmon out of the fridge, place it on preheated grill over medium-high heat and cook it for 3 minutes.

Flip salmon, cook for 3 more minutes and divide on serving plates. Top each salmon piece with avocado sauce and serve.

Shrimp With Mango and Avocado Mix

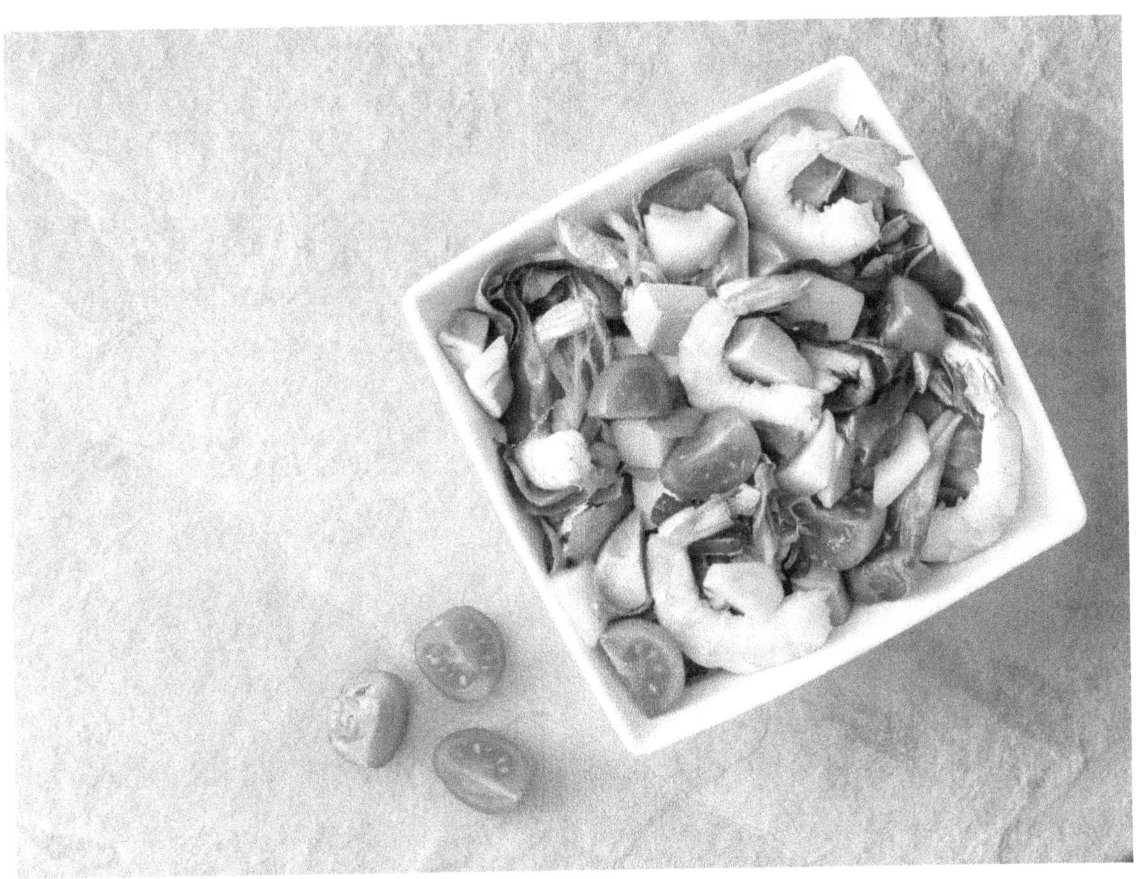

I'm sure you're familiar with shrimp and avocado. Well, these two ingredients are a match made in paradise when paired together in a gorgeous dip. Super delicious and healthy, this dip is an absolute must. The best part about this recipe? The avocado is blended right into the mango sauce for extra creaminess and richness!

Serving size: 2

Cooking time: 8 minutes

Ingredients:

- 1 avocado pitted, peeled and chopped
- 1 lb. shrimp peeled and deveined
- 1 tomato chopped
- 1 mango peeled and chopped
- 1 jalapeno chopped
- 1 tbsp. lime juice
- Bacon fat
- ¼ cup green onions, chopped
- 4 garlic cloves, minced
- A pinch of sea salt
- Black pepper to the taste

Instructions:

In a bowl, mix lime juice with jalapeno, mango, tomato, avocado, and green onions, stir well and leave aside.

Heat a pan with some bacon fat over medium-high heat, add garlic, stir and cook for 2 minutes.

Add shrimp, a pinch of sea salt and black pepper, stir, and cook for 5 minutes. Divide shrimp on plates, add mango and avocado mix on the side.

Fish Dish

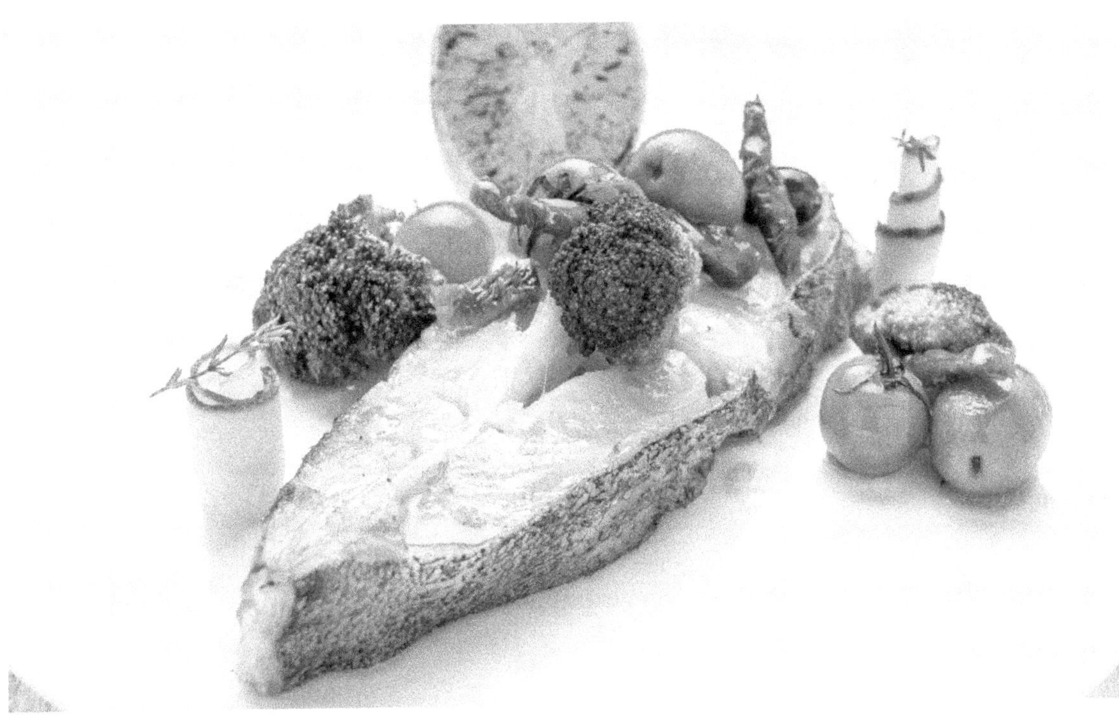

It can be boiled, fried, grilled, or even smoked– and you can eat it for breakfast or dinner. The rich flavor that fish has is a perfect complement to almost any type of cuisine- while some people like it served with simple sauces such as lemon and parsley butter sauce, others like it served with more complex sauces such as curry sauce.

Serving size: 4

Cooking time: 15 minutes

Ingredients:

- ¼ cup ghee; melted
- 4 halibut fish fillets
- 4 garlic cloves; minced
- 2 tbsp. parsley; chopped
- Zest and juice from 1 lemon
- 1 lemon; sliced
- A pinch of sea salt
- Black pepper to the taste

Instructions:

In a bowl mix, garlic with ghee, lemon zest, juice, parsley, a pinch of sea salt and pepper, and stir well.

Arrange fish in a baking dish, season with pepper to the taste, drizzle the mix you've made, top with lemon slices, introduce in the oven at 425°F and bake for 15 minutes. Divide between plates and serve warm.

Shrimp Dish

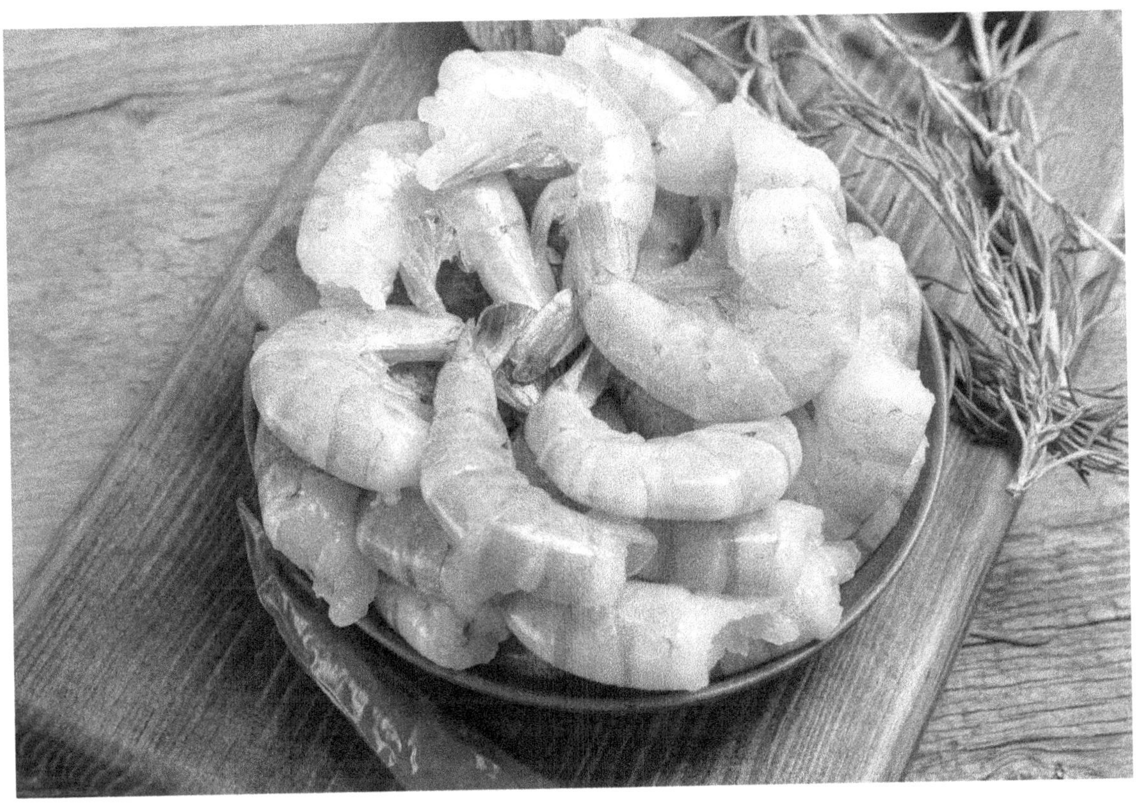

It is a straightforward, quick, and yummy dish that you can make in no time! What makes shrimp a favorite food is its light and delicate taste. In addition, shrimp can also be prepared many different ways and with several other ingredients.

Serving size: 4

Cooking time: 8 minutes

Ingredients:

- 20 shrimp; peeled and deveined
- 1 chopped medium red bell pepper
- 1 chopped medium yellow onion
- 1 finely chopped garlic clove
- 5 dried red chilies
- ¼ cup coconut aminos
- 1 inch ginger, minced
- ¼ tsp. sea salt
- 2 tbsp. coconut oil
- ¼ tsp. Black pepper
- 2 tbsp. water
- 1 tsp. apple cider vinegar
- 1 tbsp. lime juice
- 1 tsp. raw honey
- A handful cilantro; finely chopped for serving

Instructions:

In a bowl, mix aminos with lime juice, water, vinegar, and honey and whisk well.

Over medium heat, heat coconut oil in a pan. Add ginger and garlic, stir and cook for about 2 minutes.

Add bell pepper, red chilies, onion, stir and cook for additional 4 minutes.

Add shrimp, a pinch of salt and pepper to the taste. Add vinegar mix, stir and cook for 5 minutes.

Serve and top with cilantro.

Roasted Trout

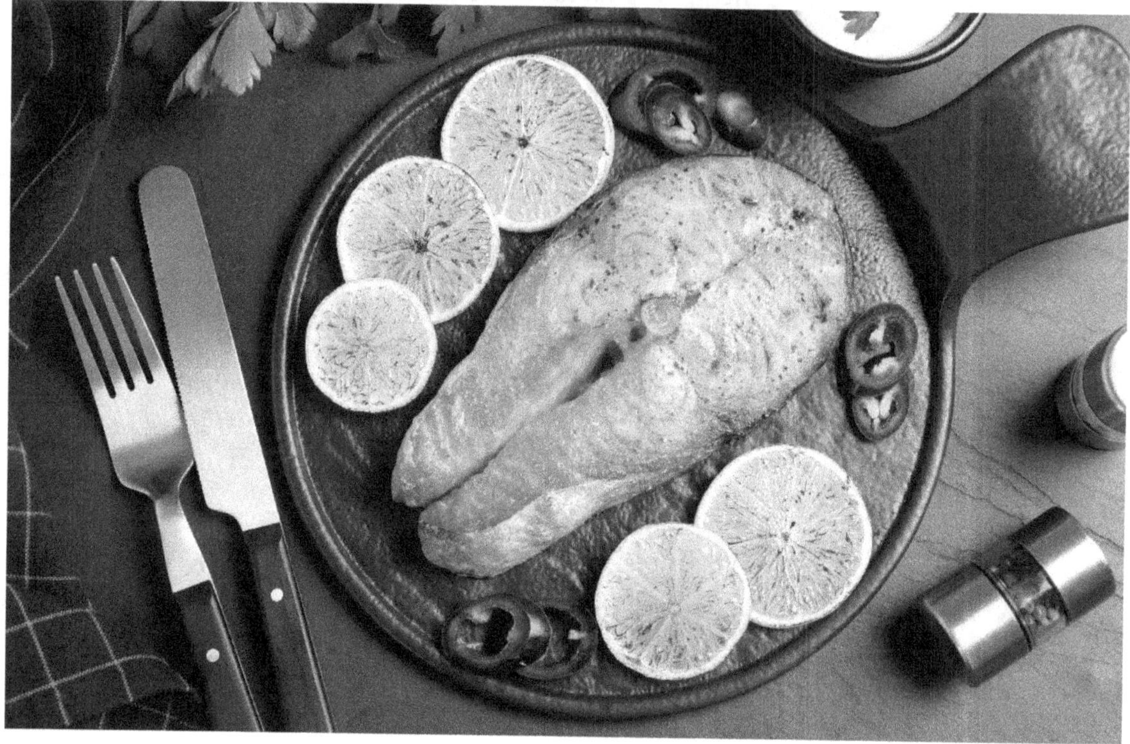

Roasted trout is a delicious, healthy, and easy-to-prepare fish. It's quick to cook, and it tastes great. Its flesh is orange and flaky, with a mild, delicate flavor similar to that of salmon or mackerel. It's not as oily as those types of fish either; trout has few calories compared with other types of meat because it doesn't have any fat on its body.

Serving size: 4

Cooking time: 22 minutes

Ingredients:

- 3 trout; cleaned and gutted
- 1 bunch dill
- 2 lemons; sliced
- 1 bunch rosemary
- 2 fennel bulbs; sliced
- A pinch of sea salt
- Black pepper to the taste
- 2 tbsp. extra virgin olive oil

Instructions:

Grease a baking dish with some oil, spread fennel slices on the bottom, and add trout after you've seasoned them with a pinch of sea salt and pepper.

Fill each fish with lemon slices, dill, and rosemary springs.

Top fish with the rest of the herbs and lemon slices, drizzle the rest of the oil, introduce everything in the oven at 500°F and bake for 10 minutes.

Reduce heat to 425°F and bake for 12 more minutes. Leave fish to cool down, divide between plates and serve.

Salmon and Tomato Pesto

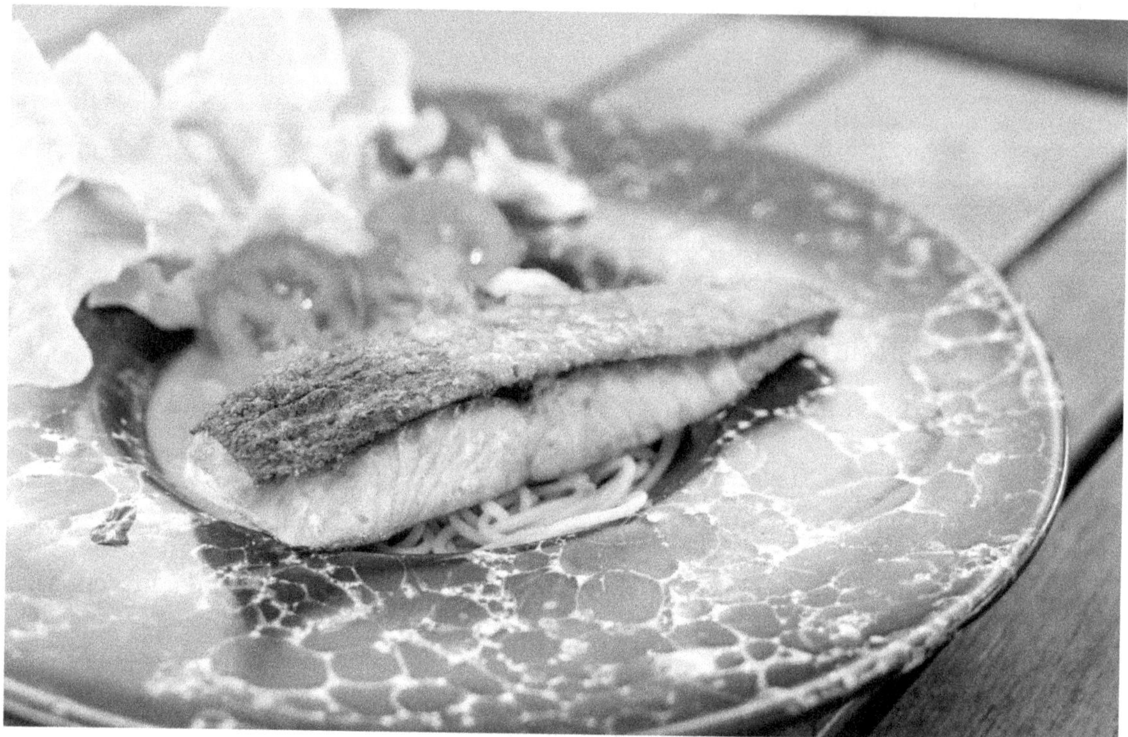

When it comes to pesto, salmon and tomatoes are the perfect duos. They're rich sources of protein while providing a light, fresh flavor. It's simple to make with ingredients you may already have in your kitchen! This pesto has a bright acidity from lemon juice that balances the richness of the Parmesan cheese.

Serving size: 4

Cooking time: 12 minutes

Ingredients:

- 4 salmon fillets; skin on
- 1 tbsp. red bell pepper; chopped
- 1 shallot; chopped
- 2 tbsp. basil; chopped
- ½ cup cherry tomatoes; cut in quarters
- 2 garlic cloves; minced
- ½ cup sun-dried tomatoes; chopped
- 3 tbsp. olive oil
- A pinch of sea salt
- Black pepper to the taste

Instructions:

In your food processor, mix sun-dried tomatoes with garlic, oil, basil, shallots, a pinch of sea salt, and black pepper and blend well.

Rub salmon with some of this mix, place on preheated grill over medium-high heat, cook for 12 minutes, flipping once and divide between plates. Add the rest of the tomato pesto on top and serve with cherry tomatoes and bell pepper pieces on the side.

Cod And Herb Sauce

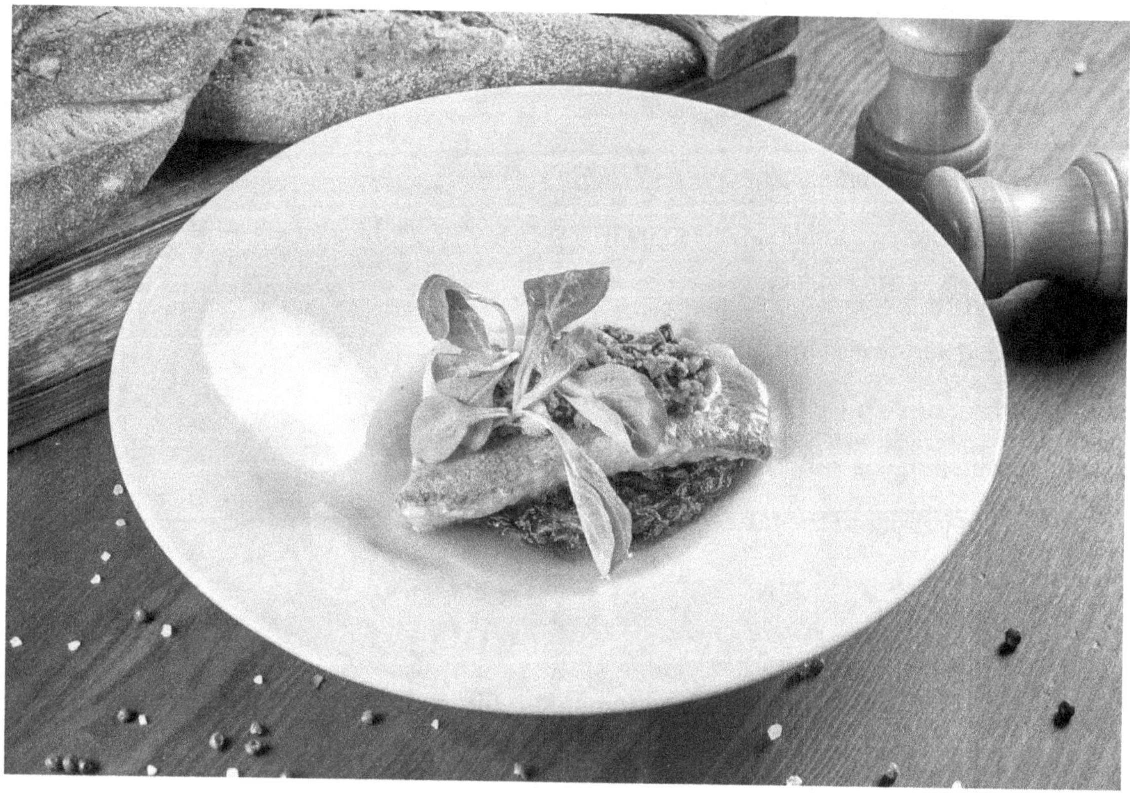

The Cod and Herb sauce is made from white fish in an herb and olive oil sauce. This meal typically includes rice as a starch, but it can also be served with pasta if desired. It is accompanied by Parmesan cheese or other cheeses to top it off.

Serving size: 4

Cooking time: 16 minutes

Ingredients:

- 1 tbsp. chives; chopped
- 4 medium cod fillets
- 1 tbsp. thymc; chopped
- 1 tbsp. parsley; chopped
- Grated zest from ½ lemon
- 1 shallot; chopped
- 3/4 cup coconut milk
- 6 tbsp. ghee
- 2 garlic cloves
- A pinch of sea salt
- Black pepper to the taste

Instructions:

In a bowl, mix garlic with ghee, shallots, chives, parsley, and thyme and stir well.

Season cod with a pinch of salt and black pepper to the taste.

Heat a pan over medium heat, add herbed ghee and fish, toss to coat, and cook for 2 minutes on each side.

Transfer fish to a lined baking sheet, place in the oven at 400°F, and bake for 7 minutes.

Heat the pan with the herbed ghee over medium heat, add lemon zest and coconut milk, stir and bring to a simmer over medium heat. Divide fish on plates, drizzle the herbed sauce on top, and serve.

Chapter 4: Vegetable recipes

Stuffed Zucchinis

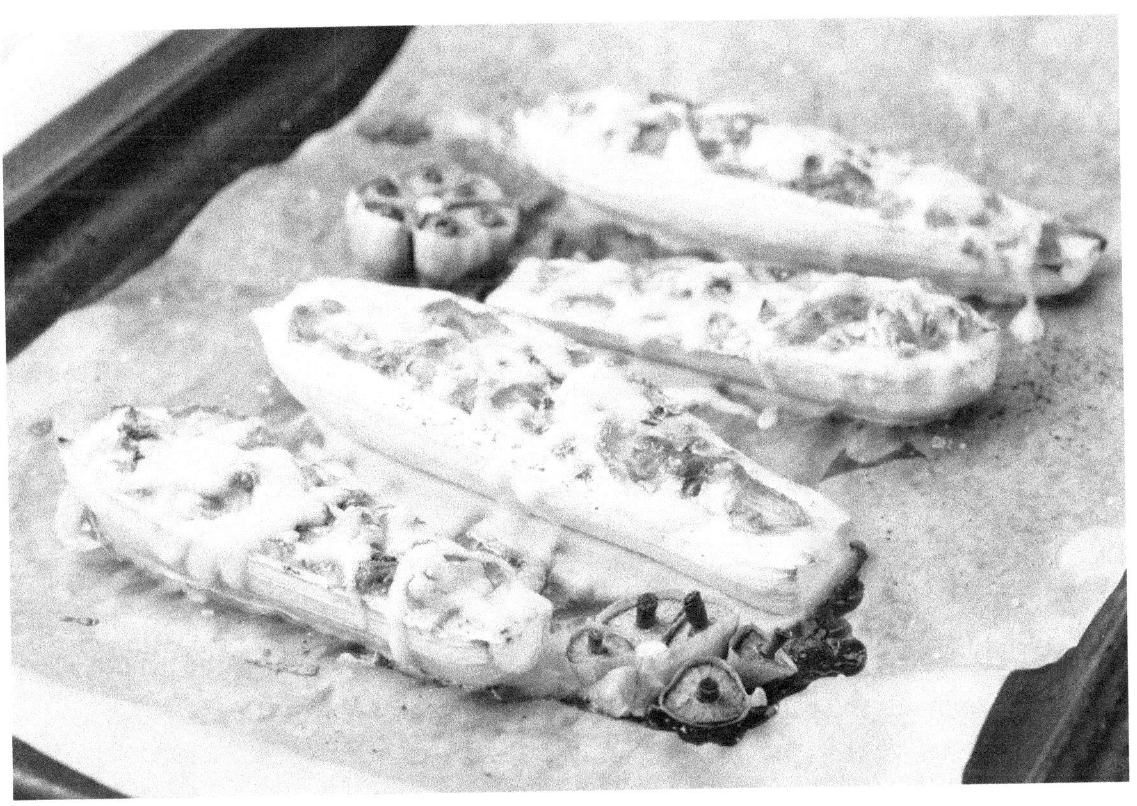

Stuffed zucchinis are an easy way to get a low-carb, high-protein meal that will make you forget about meat! The perfect dish for vegetarians and those who are trying to lower their cholesterol.

Zucchini is a type of squash that can be eaten raw or cooked. They come in various lengths, thicknesses, and colors which makes them perfect containers for stuffing with your favorite ingredients.

Serving size: 4

Cooking time: 20 minutes

Ingredients:

- 2 tomatoes; chopped
- 1 eggplant; chopped
- 2 zucchinis; cut into halves lengthwise
- 1 yellow onion; chopped
- A pinch of sea salt
- Black pepper to the taste
- ½ bunch parsley; finely chopped
- 3 tbsp. extra virgin olive oil
- 2 garlic cloves; minced

Instructions:

Remove flesh from zucchini halves, season them with a pinch of sea salt and pepper, leave aside for 10 minutes and pat dry them,

Heat a pan with 1 tbsp. oil over medium high heat, add onion, stir and cook for 4 minutes.

Add garlic, stir and cook 1 minute. Add the rest of the oil, eggplant and chopped zucchini flesh, stir and cook for 10 minutes.

Add tomatoes, parsley and pepper to the taste, stir and cook for 5 minutes more.

Fill zucchini halves with this mix, place on preheated grill over medium high heat, cook for 3 minutes, and divide between plates and serve right away.

Broccoli And Cauliflower Fritters

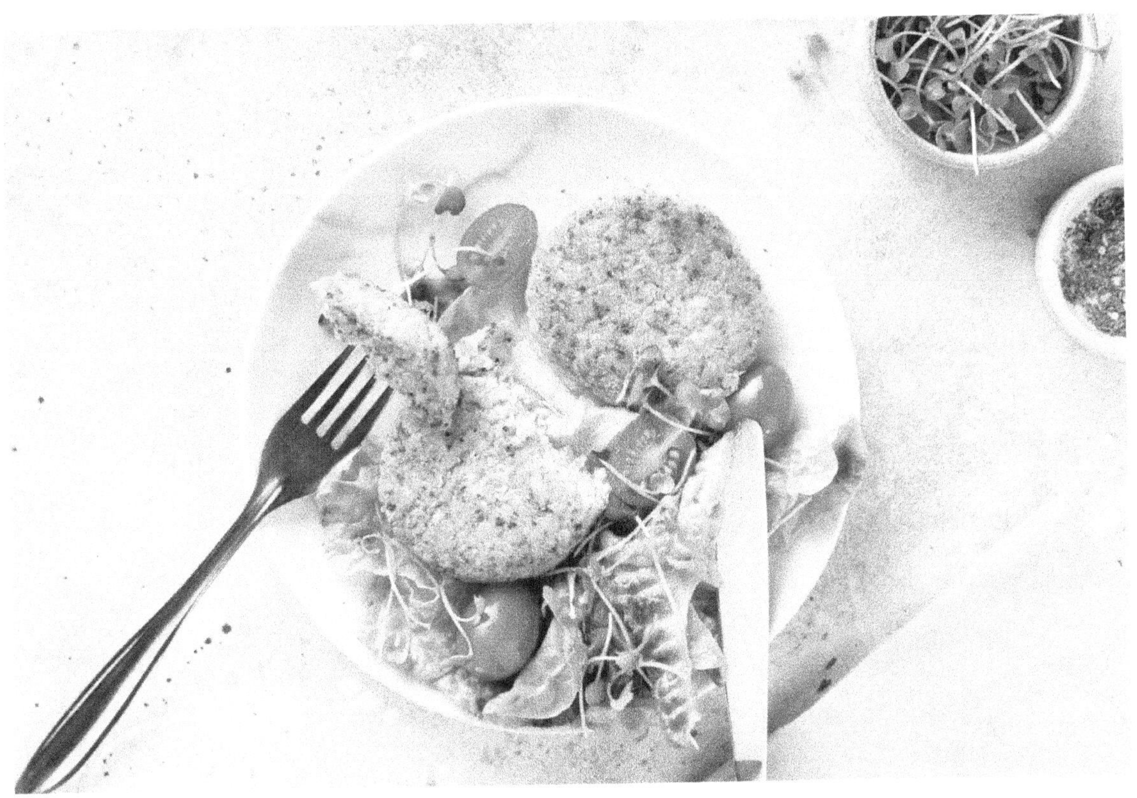

Broccoli and cauliflower fritters are the perfect way to incorporate vegetables into your diet. They're easy, fast, and can be made vegan or gluten-free!

It's been shown that eating more vegetables can have a tremendous impact on one's health. It helps weight loss, reduces symptoms of chronic disease such as diabetes and cancer, improves mental clarity - the list goes on.

Serving size: 8

Cooking time: 4 minutes

Ingredients:

- 1 cup broccoli, chopped
- 1½ cups cauliflower chopped
- A pinch of sea salt
- Black pepper to the taste
- 1 tbsp. coconut flour
- 2 eggs
- 1 tbsp. coconut oil for frying
- 2 tbsp. homemade mayonnaise
- 1 tbsp. extra virgin olive oil
- 1 tbsp. coriander, finely chopped
- ½ garlic clove; grated
- 1 tsp. lime juice

Instructions:

In a bowl, mix cauliflower with broccoli, eggs, coconut flour, a pinch of sea salt and pepper to the taste and stir very well.

Shape small patties and arrange them on a plate.

Heat a pan with the coconut oil over medium-high heat, add veggies fritters, cook for 4 minutes on each side, transfer them to paper towels, drain grease and arrange on a platter.

In a bowl, mix mayo with olive oil, coriander, garlic, and lime juice and stir well.

Serve your fritters with mayo mix.

Stuffed Eggplant

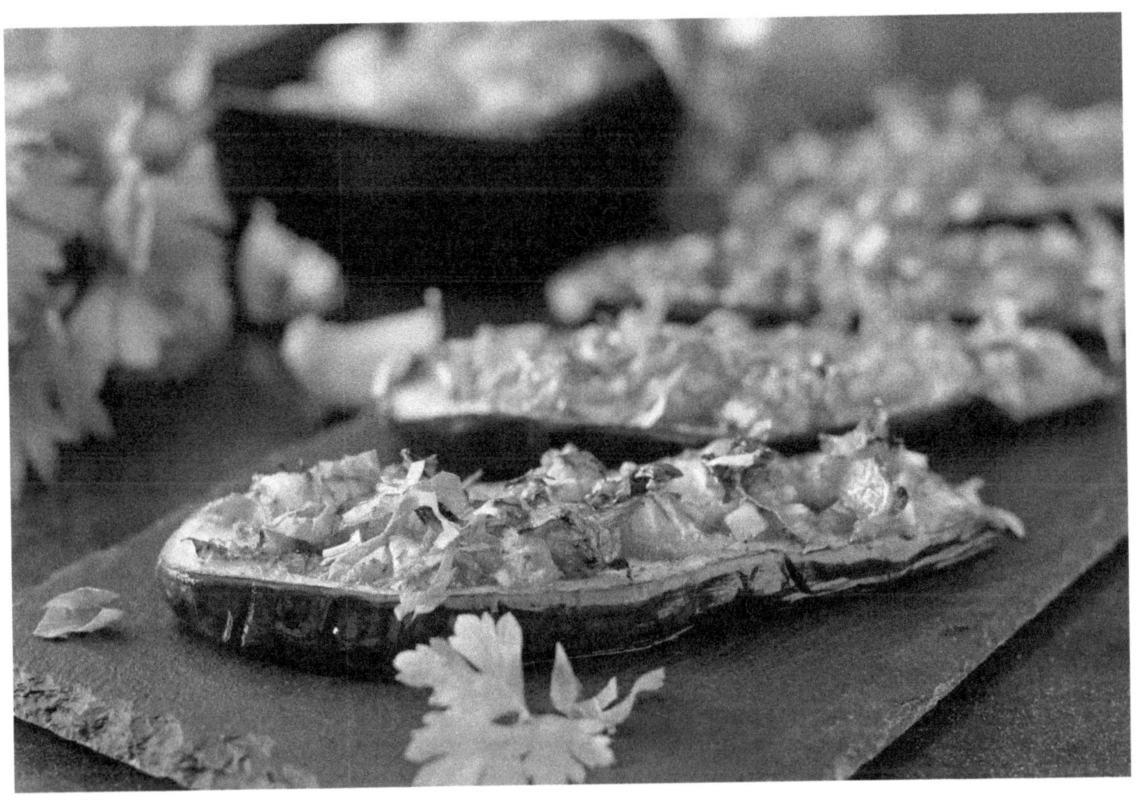

You know those meals that you cook time and time again because they're so easy and delicious? Stuffed eggplant is one of them.

This dish is an old classic, made by stuffing a halved eggplant with a mix of tomatoes, garlic, breadcrumbs, salt, and pepper.

Serving size: 2

Cooking time: 55 minutes

Ingredients:

- 1 eggplant
- 2 tomatoes; finely chopped
- 3 thyme springs
- 1 garlic clove; minced
- 3 tbsp. extra virgin olive oil
- A pinch of sea salt
- Black pepper to the taste
- Lemon juice from ½ lemon

Instructions:

Place eggplant on a lined baking sheet, introduce in the oven at 400°F and bake for 30 minutes.

Take the eggplant out of the oven, leave aside to cool down, cut in half lengthways, drizzle each half with 1 tbsp. olive oil, introduce in the oven again at 350°F, and bake for 25 more minutes.

Take eggplant halves out of the oven, leave aside for 5 minutes, discard the flesh and sprinkle halves with some lemon juice, a pinch of sea salt and pepper.

In a bowl, mix tomatoes with thyme, garlic, and chopped eggplant flesh and stir.

Add lemon juice, pepper, and 1 tbsp. olive oil and stir everything well. Scoop this into eggplant halves, divide on a plate and serve.

Veggies and Fish Mix

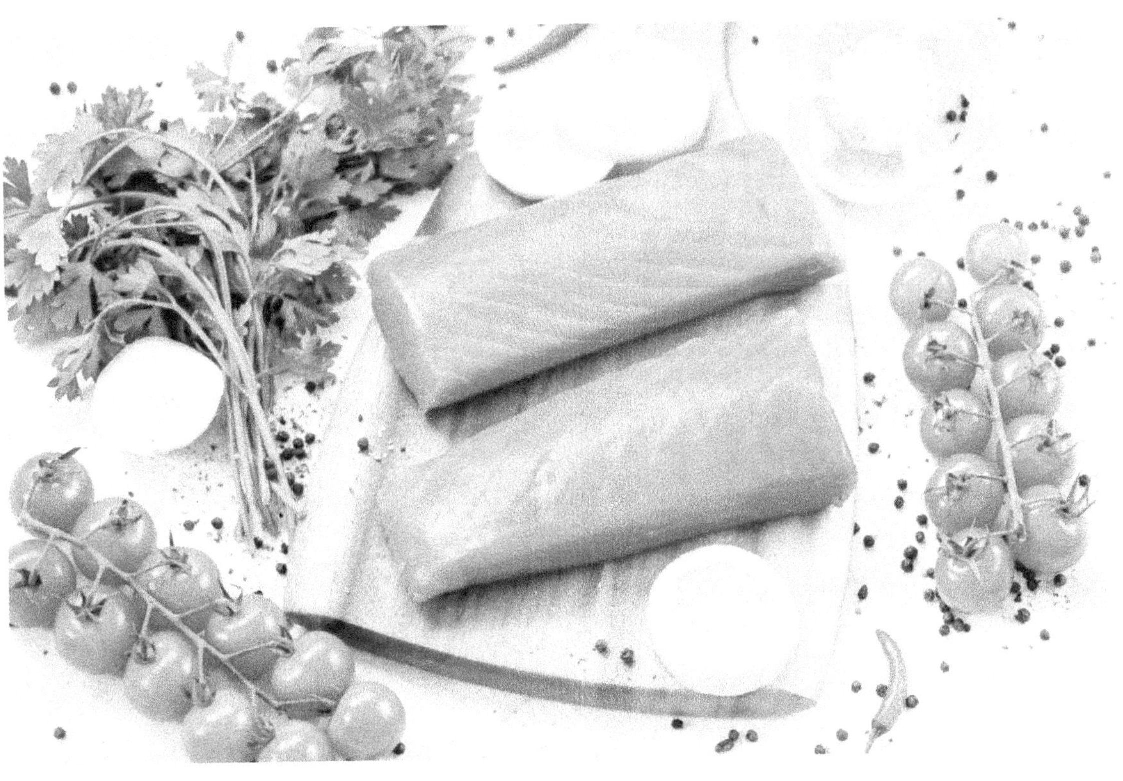

Did you know that fried veggies and fish is one of the best recipes for kids? With a few other ingredients, your child can create a great meal like this. Plus, it is easy to make and takes less than 10 minutes. So get creative with your loved ones- let them know how much you appreciate all they do!

Serving size: 4

Cooking time: 32 minutes

Ingredients:

- 1 cup hot water
- 1 tbsp. maple syrup
- 2 tbsp. olive oil
- 1 eggplant; chopped
- 3 cups cherry tomatoes; halved
- 1 tsp. Tabasco sauce
- 1 lb. tuna; cubed
- 1 tsp. balsamic vinegar
- ½ cup basil; chopped
- Black pepper to the taste
- A pinch of sea salt

Instructions:

In a bowl, mix eggplant pieces with a pinch of salt and black pepper and stir.

Heat a pan with 1 tbsp. oil over medium heat, add eggplant, cook for 6 minutes, and transfer to a bowl.

Heat the pan again with the rest of the oil over medium heat, add tomatoes, cover pan and cook for 6 minutes, shaking the pan from time to time.

Return eggplant pieces to the pan, add maple syrup, vinegar, and hot water, stir; cover, and cook for 10 minutes.

Add tuna and Tabasco sauce, stir; cover pan again, reduce heat to medium-low and simmer for 10 minutes more. Sprinkle basil on top, divide veggies and tuna mix between plates and serve.

Veggies Dish with Tasty Sauce

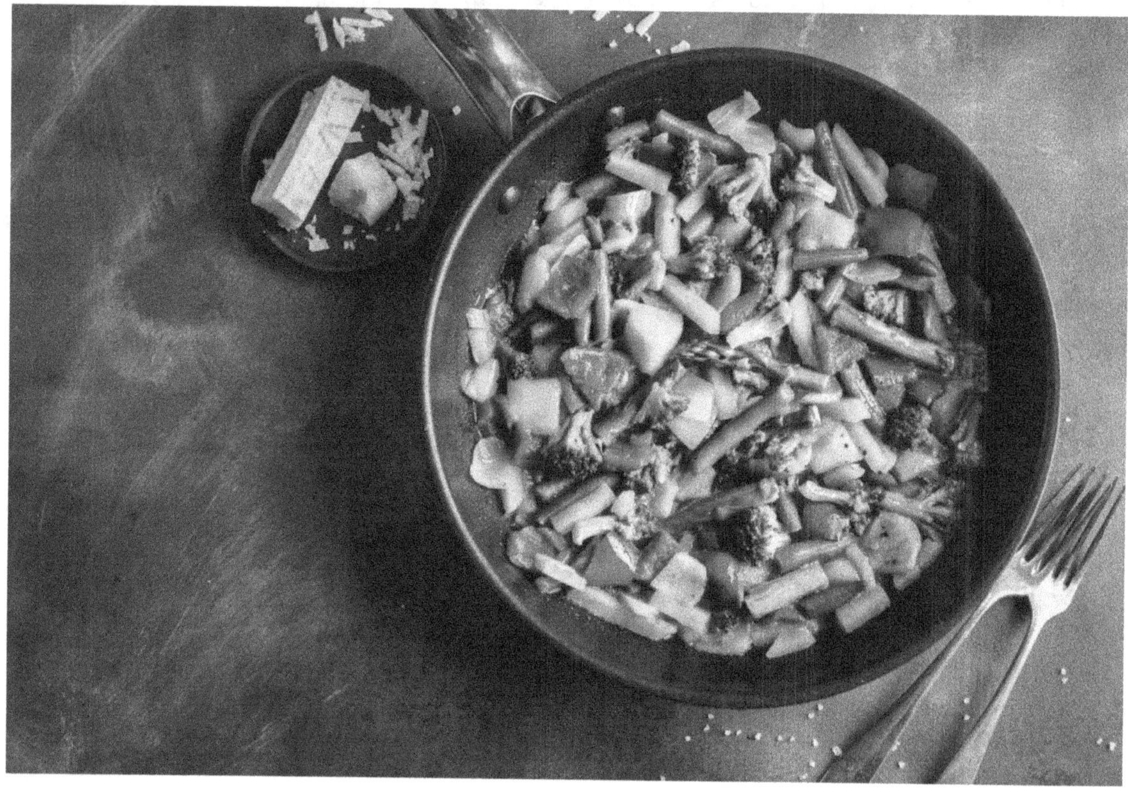

Are you tired of the same old boring vegetables for dinner? Well, we have just the recipe for you! This dish has a delicious creamy sauce that will blow you away with its flavor.

Serving size: 4

Cooking time: 12 minutes

Ingredients:

- 2 carrots; chopped
- 8 mushrooms; sliced
- 4 zucchinis; cut in thin noodles
- 2 cups spinach; torn
- 2 yellow squash; halved and sliced
- 1 tbsp. coconut oil
- 1 cup coconut milk
- Juice of 1 lemon
- A pinch of sea salt
- Black pepper to the taste

For the pesto:

- ½ cup extra virgin olive oil
- 2 cups basil
- 1/3 cup pine nuts
- 3 garlic clove; chopped
- A pinch of sea salt
- Black pepper to the taste

Instructions:

In your food processor, mix basil with nuts and garlic and pulse well.

Add oil, a pinch of salt and pepper, pulse well again, transfer to a bowl and leave aside.

Steam carrots, squash, zucchini and mushrooms in a bamboo steamer for 8 minutes, transfer them to a colander, season with a pinch of sea salt and pepper, leave aside for 10 minutes, pat dry them and put in a bowl.

Heat up a pan with the oil over medium-high heat, add half of the coconut milk, salt and pepper and bring to a boil stirring all the time.

Add the pesto you've made, lemon juice and the rest of the coconut milk and stir again.

Add steamed veggies, stir and cook for 2 minutes. Add spinach, more salt and pepper if needed, stir; cook for 2 minutes more, transfer to bowls and serve.

Bell Peppers Stuffed with Tuna

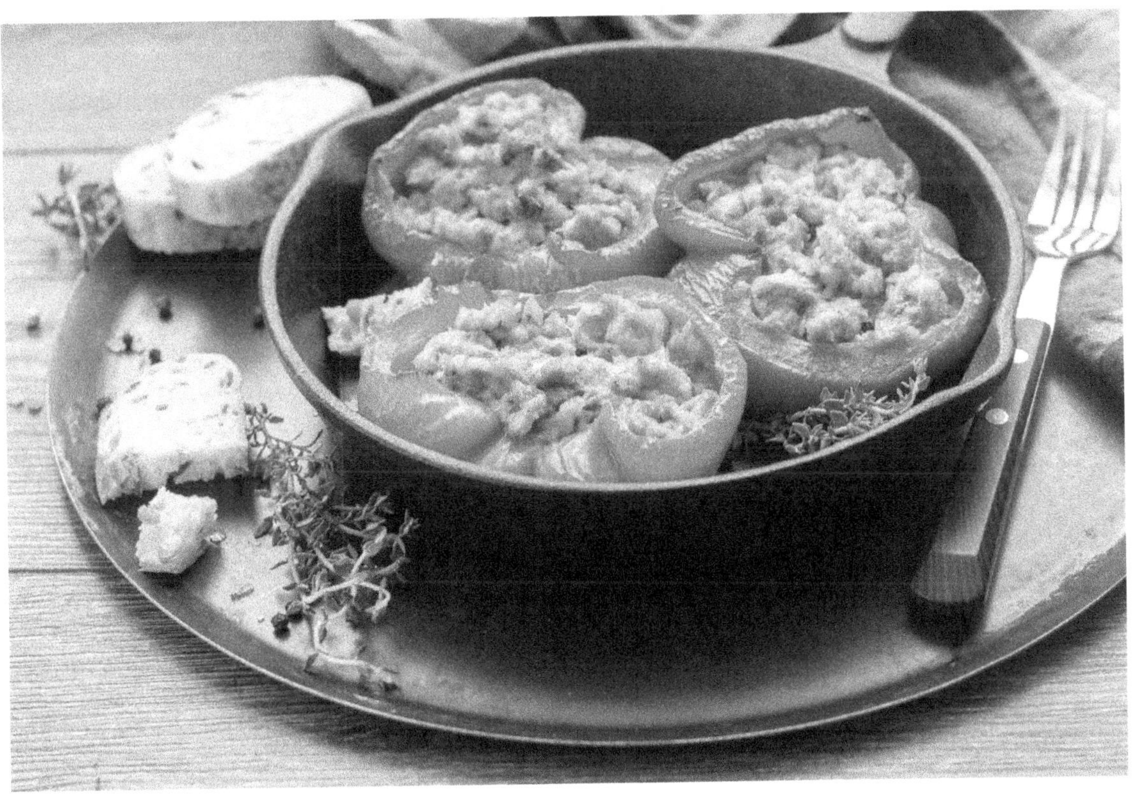

Bell peppers stuffed with tuna and a garlic-sherry sauce are easy to make for a simple weeknight meal. This dish is low in calories but high in vitamins, fiber, and protein. It's perfect for making ahead of time or for taking along as part of a healthy lunch.

Serving size: 4

Cooking time: 10 minutes

Ingredients:

- 2 bell peppers; tops cut off, cut in halves and seeds removed
- 1 tbsp. capers; chopped
- 2 tbsp. tomato puree
- 4 oz. canned tuna; drained and flaked
- 1 scallion; chopped
- 1 tomato; chopped
- Black pepper to the taste

Instructions:

Place bell pepper halves on a lined baking sheet, place in preheated broiler over medium-high heat, boil for 4 minutes and then leave them aside to cool down.

Meanwhile, in a bowl, mix capers with tomato puree, tuna, tomato, black pepper, and scallion and stir well.

Stuff bell peppers with this mix, place in preheated broiler again, and cook for 5 minutes. Divide between plates and serve.

Eggplant Dish

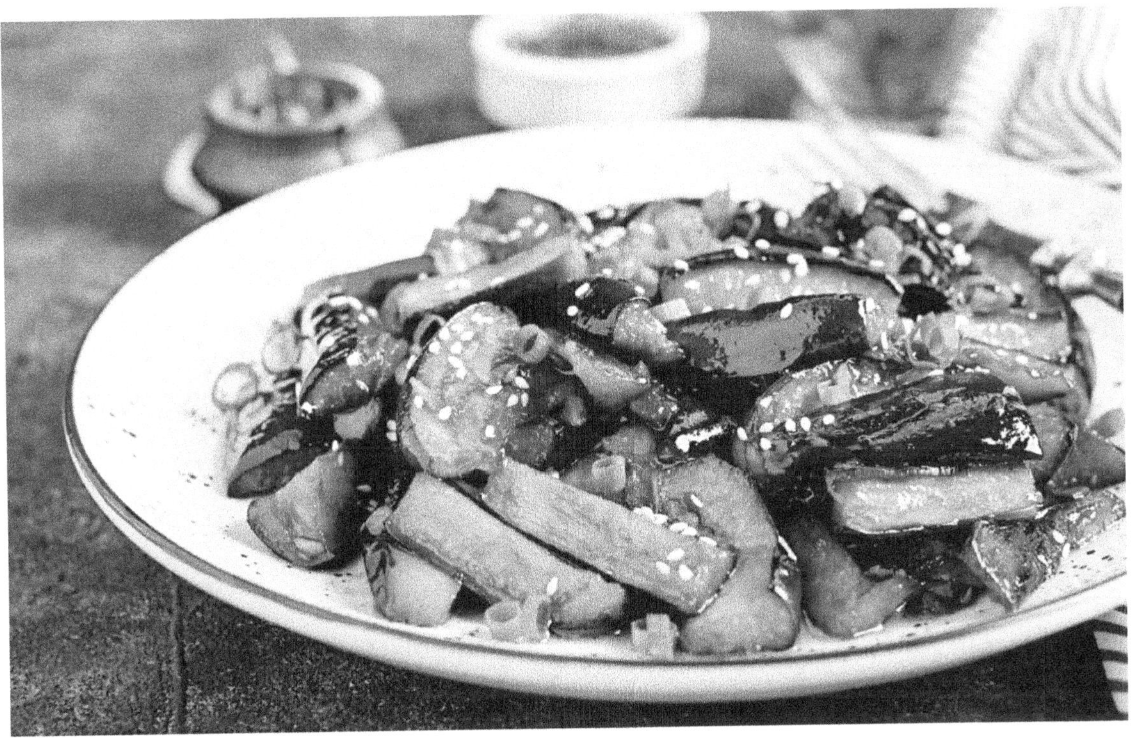

This dish is a perfect side for any meal and can be used as the main dish if desired! Eggplant is one of my favorite veggies. Its creamy texture goes well with any sauce. You can add some zucchini to make it more filling. An easy way to cook eggplant, this recipe is quick and simple. The vegetables will all cook at once, so no need to prep them before cooking.

Serving size: 3

Cooking time: 40 minutes

Ingredients:

- 5 medium eggplants; sliced into rounds
- 1 tsp. thyme; chopped
- 2 tbsp. balsamic vinegar
- 1 tsp. mustard
- 2 garlic cloves; minced
- ½ cup olive oil
- Black pepper to the taste
- A pinch of sea salt
- 1 tsp. maple syrup

Instructions:

In a bowl, mix vinegar with thyme, mustard, garlic, oil, salt, pepper and maple syrup and whisk very well.

Arrange eggplant round on a lined baking sheet, place in the oven at 425°F and roast for 40 minutes. Divide eggplants between plates and serve.

Zucchini Noodles and Capers Sauce

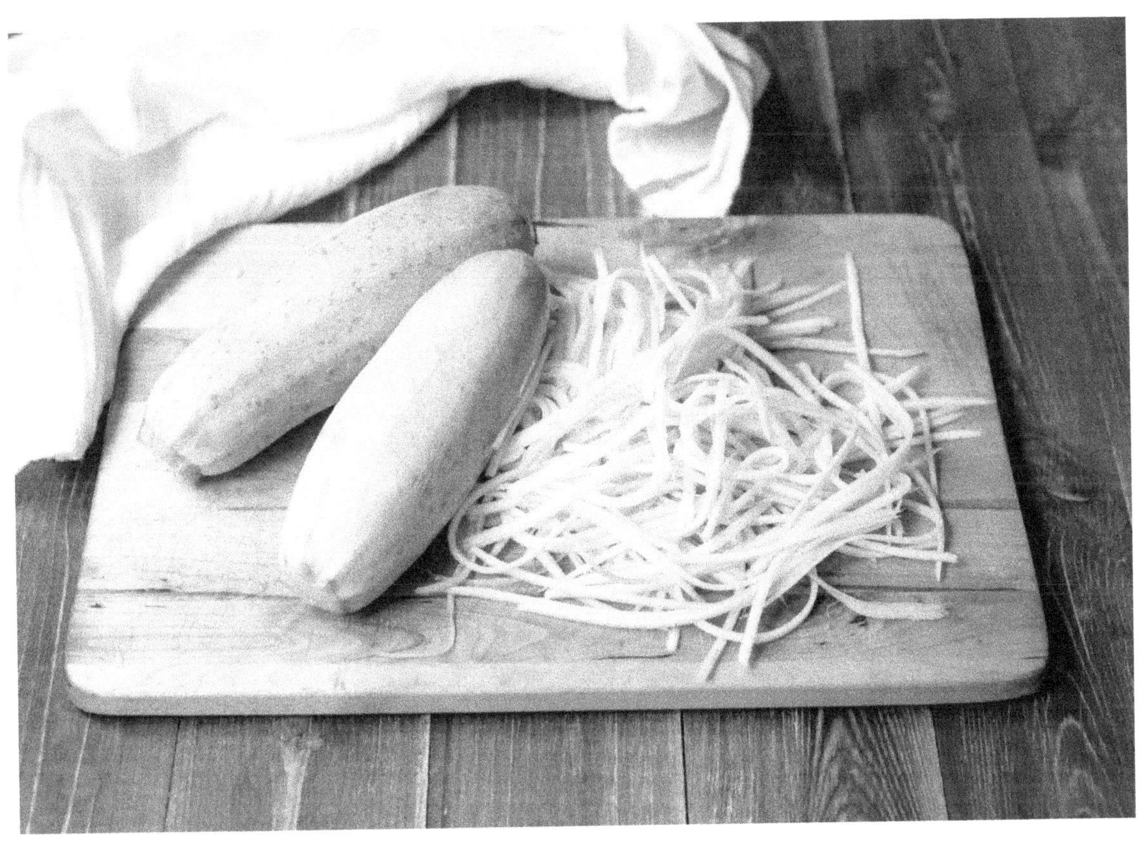

With this dish, made with zucchini noodles and capers sauce, you can have your favorite Italian food without guilt. Not only is this meal delicious and hearty, but it's also super easy to make!

This dish looks great as a meatless option for dinner or when you're looking for something light.

Serving size: 4

Cooking time: 10 minutes

Ingredients:

- 1 tbsp. capers; drained
- 1 garlic clove
- A pinch of sea salt
- Black pepper to the taste
- A pinch of red pepper flakes
- 15 kalamata olives; pitted
- 2 tbsp. olive oil
- 8 oz. cherry tomatoes; halved
- A handful basil; torn
- Juice of ½ lemon
- 4 zucchinis; cut with a spiralizer

Instructions:

In your food processor, mix capers with a pinch of sea salt, black pepper, pepper flakes and olives and blend well.

Transfer this to a bowl add basil, oil and tomatoes, stir well and leave aside for 10 minutes. Divide zucchini noodles on plates, add tomatoes and capers sauce, toss to coat well and serve.

Sweet Potatoes and Cabbage Bake

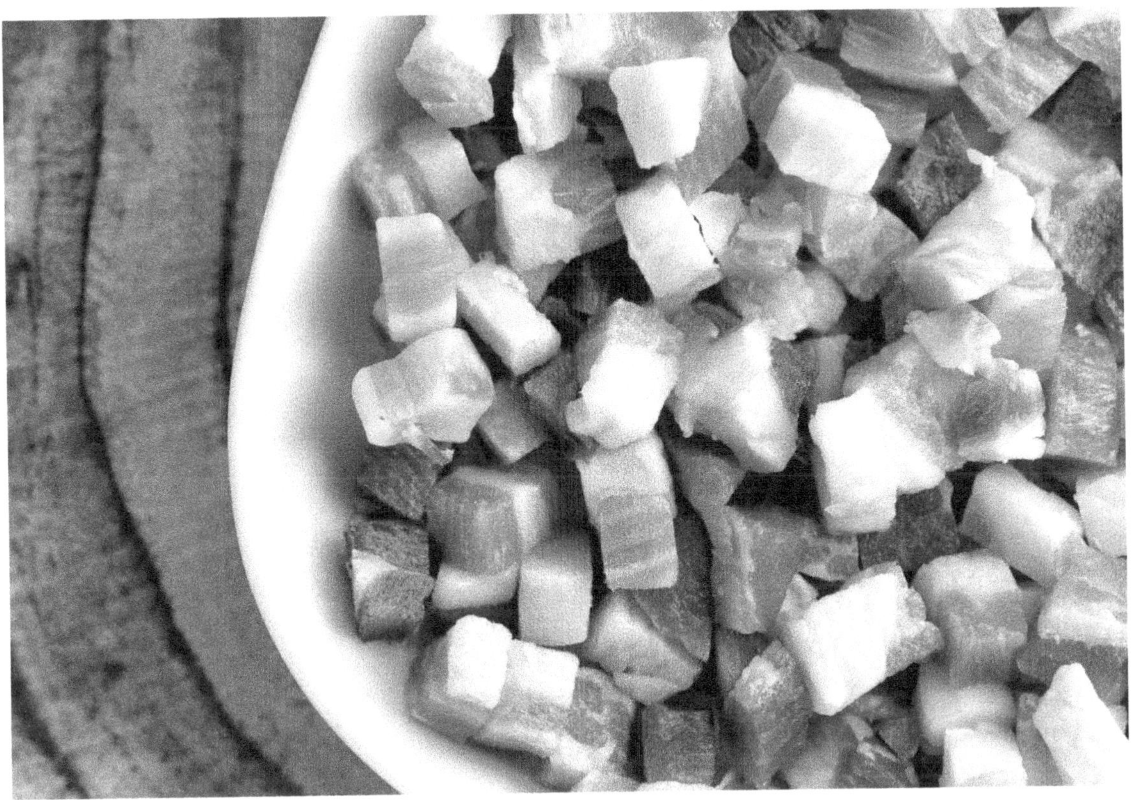

This sweet potato and cabbage recipe makes a delicious, healthy side dish or vegetarian casserole. It can be eaten hot or cold and is very low in calories. Sweet potatoes are a type of root vegetable high in beta-carotene and vitamin A. They contain antioxidants that can help fight the free radicals in our bodies to keep us healthy.

Serving size: 4

Cooking time: 1 hour 5 minutes

Ingredients:

- 8 sweet potatoes; cut into thin matchsticks
- 1 carrot; sliced
- 2½ cups green cabbage; shredded
- 2 garlic cloves; minced
- A pinch of sea salt
- Black pepper to the taste
- 4 oz. pancetta; chopped
- 3 tomatoes; sliced
- 1 tsp. thyme; dried

Instructions:

In a baking dish, mix cabbage with potatoes, garlic and carrot.

Add thyme, a pinch of sea salt and pepper and pancetta and toss to coat.

Spread tomato slices over veggie mix, cover dish with tin foil, introduce in the oven at 350°F and bake for 35 minutes.

Discard tin foil and bake veggies for 30 more minutes. Take the dish out of the oven, leave aside to cool down, divide between plates and serve.

Stuffed Portobello Mushrooms

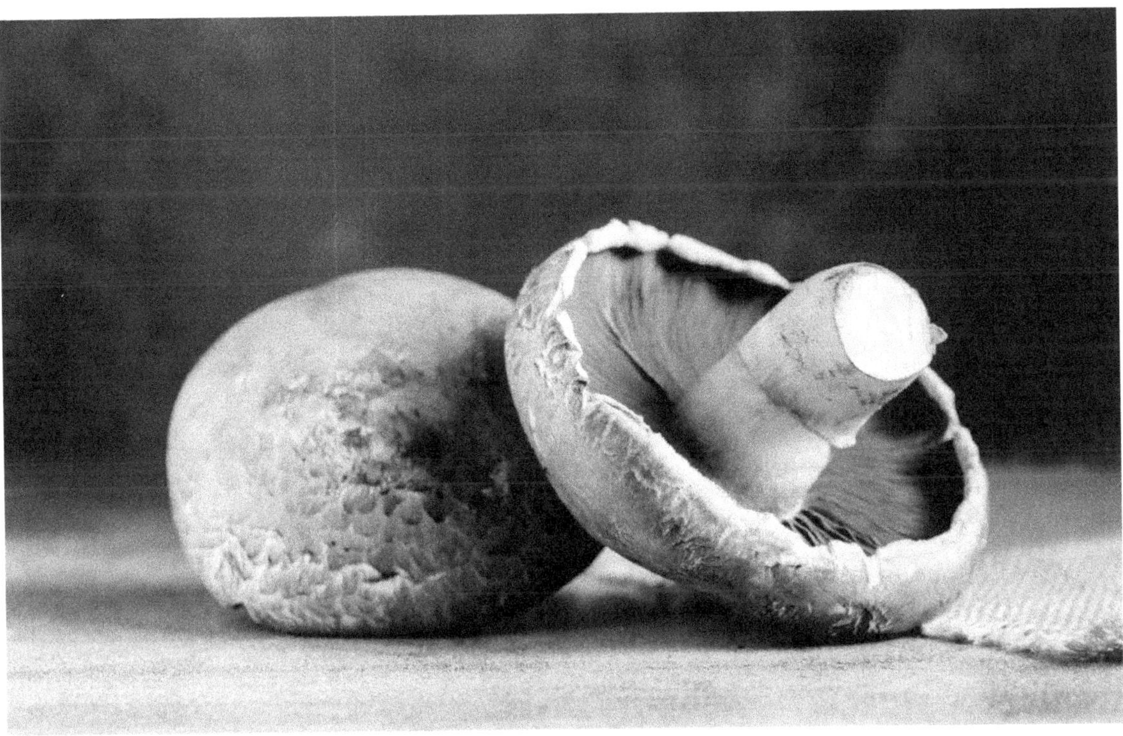

They taste good, they're nutritious, and they're always in season!

If you've ever craved a big, juicy steak but don't get the satisfaction of biting into it due to your vegetarian diet, this recipe is for you. For those who don't know, these mushrooms are large caps of Portobello mushrooms that have been hollowed out and filled with a potato and vegetable mixture that tastes like steak.

Serving size: 4

Cooking time: 20 minutes

Ingredients:

- 10 basil leaves
- 1 cup baby spinach
- 3 garlic cloves; chopped
- 1 cup almonds; roughly chopped
- 1 tbsp. parsley
- 2 tbsp. Nutritional yeast
- ¼ cup olive oil
- 8 cherry tomatoes; halved
- A pinch of sea salt
- Black pepper to the taste
- 4 Portobello mushrooms; stem removed and chopped

Instructions:

In your food processor, mix basil with spinach, garlic, almonds, parsley, Nutritional yeast, oil, a pinch of salt, black pepper to the taste and mushroom stems and blend well.

Stuff each mushroom with this mix, place them on a lined baking sheet, place in the oven at 400°F and bake for 20 minutes. Divide between plates and serve right away.

Conclusion

Thank you for getting to the end of this book. I hope you have been able to learn how to prepare lactogenic diet recipes. Just know that you are not only limited to the recipes in this book; keep exploring to get more recipes.

Happy cooking!

About the Author

Ivy's mission is to share her recipes with the world. Even though she is not a professional cook she has always had that flair toward cooking. Her hands create magic. She can make even the simplest recipe tastes superb. Everyone who has tried her food has astounding their compliments was what made her think about writing recipes.

She wanted everyone to have a taste of her creations aside from close family and friends. So, deciding to write recipes was her winning decision. She isn't interested in popularity, but how many people have her recipes reached and touched people. Each recipe in her cookbooks is special and has a special meaning in her life. This means that each recipe is created with attention and love. Every ingredient carefully picked, every combination tried and tested.

Her mission started on her birthday about 9 years ago, when her guests couldn't stop prizing the food on the table. The next thing she did was organizing an event where chefs from restaurants were tasting her recipes. This event gave her the courage to start spreading her recipes.

She has written many cookbooks and she is still working on more. There is no end in the art of cooking; all you need is inspiration, love, and dedication.

Author's Afterthoughts

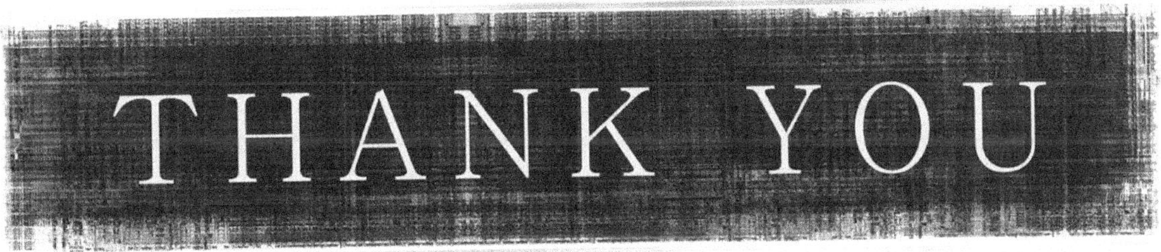

I am thankful for downloading this book and taking the time to read it. I know that you have learned a lot and you had a great time reading it. Writing books is the best way to share the skills I have with your and the best tips too.

I know that there are many books and choosing my book is amazing. I am thankful that you stopped and took time to decide. You made a great decision and I am sure that you enjoyed it.

I will be even happier if you provide honest feedback about my book. Feedbacks helped by growing and they still do. They help me to choose better content and new ideas. So, maybe your feedback can trigger an idea for my next book.

Thank you again

Sincerely

Ivy Hope

www.ingramcontent.com/pod-product-compliance
Lightning Source LLC
Chambersburg PA
CBHW081836250726

48659CB00008B/2481